Management of Type 2 Diabetes Mellitus in Primary Care:
a practical guide

L. Steven Levene
General Practitioner, Leicester, UK

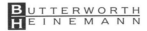

BUTTERWORTH
HEINEMANN

EDINBURGH LONDON NEW YORK OXFORD PHILADELPHIA ST LOUIS SYDNEY TORONTO 2003

Butterworth–Heinemann
An imprint of Elsevier Science Limited

ISBN 0 7506 8780 0

British Library Cataloguing in Publication Data
A catalogue record for this book is available from the British Library.
Library of Congress Cataloging in Publication Data
A catalog record for this book is available from the Library of Congress.

Note
Medical knowledge is constantly changing. As new information becomes available, changes in treatment, procedures, equipment and the use of drugs become necessary. The author/contributors and the publishers have taken great care to ensure that the information given in this text is accurate and up to date. However, readers are strongly advised to confirm that the information, especially with regard to drug usage, complies with the latest legislation and standards of practice.

Printed in China

For Butterworth–Heinemann:
Senior Commissioning Editor: Heidi Allen
Development Editor: Robert Edwards/Kim Benson
Production Manager: Yolanta Motylinska
Design and Layout: Judith Campbell
Project Management/Copyediting: John Ormiston

The
Publisher's
policy is to use
**paper manufactured
from sustainable forests**

Contents

Foreword

The prevalence of type 2 diabetes mellitus has reached pandemic proportions. It was estimated that worldwide there were 151 million people with diabetes in 2001, over 90% of these with type 2. These figures are set to rise by close to 50% in the next decade. In the UK there are close to 1.5 million people with known diabetes and approximately another million in whom diabetes has not yet been diagnosed.

Over the years, diabetes and its problems have slowly crept up the UK health agenda. The promise of a National Service Framework (NSF) has placed diabetes centre stage, and highlighted many of the current problems in diabetes care. One of these is the shortage of health professionals; another is where should care take place?

It is obvious that in any given area or 'health economy' there needs to be provision for both 'general' diabetes care and 'specialist' care. Cleary, nurses, be they general or specialist, form an important component of the care team. Medical care comes from both specialists and GPs, and most of it should be community based, although only a minority of specialists currently work in the community setting. Obviously, GPs are key members of the team – there are over 30,000 GPs compared with fewer than 600 specialists. In addition, better, more convenient care can often be given when patients are in the familiar surroundings of their own general practice.

It is axiomatic that if a proportion of GPs is to take a special interest in diabetes, they need knowledge, practice and continuing education. This is often not available. This book fills one of the large lacunae in this educational armamentarium. It is written for GPs by a GP and ties the text into the NSF standards. It is a fund of common sense, giving good practical, organisational and clinical guidance, and is a 'must' for all GPs who run diabetes services for their patients. I would go further and suggest that it should be read by practice nurses, community podiatrists and the rest of the team also. With potentially two million plus people with diabetes to look after, we need all the help we can get!

KGMM Alberti
President, International Diabetes Federation
Professor of Medicine, University of Newcastle
Vice President, Diabetes UK

Preface

Since I began working on this book, the management of type 2 diabetes mellitus has become even more important in primary care's workload and in the government's health policy. With the recent publication of the National Service Framework and the allied National Clinical Guidelines, both our patients and the government will expect practices to deliver appropriate and effective care to a high standard.

Increasingly, health care professionals are being bombarded by new research findings, new guidelines from various learned bodies and new information about treatments. Before changing their practice, the nonspecialists who deliver the bulk of diabetic care need to assess carefully all this new information, with a shrewd awareness of any potential clinical, organisational and financial pitfalls. The gap between the targets that the expert bodies advise and/or managers expect and the reality that a stretched primary care service can deliver for each individual patient may not be bridgeable in all circumstances.

This book is aimed at all members of the primary health care team. I have concentrated throughout on providing practical advice. Greater knowledge and skills will promote the delivery of high-quality care to patients with type 2 diabetes in the community and, hopefully, reduce the impact of cardiovascular disease in this high-risk group. I believe that many of the concepts discussed in the book (e.g., improving vascular risk factors, enabling patients to self-manage, consulting effectively and using psychological techniques to influence health-related behaviour) are relevant to most patient–professional encounters. Hopefully, readers will find the following pages useful.

Steven Levene
February 2003

Acknowledgements

I thank the following professional colleagues for allowing me to 'pick their brains' about diabetes or for their comments on what I have written: George Alberti, Richard Baker, Mary Burden, Tim Coleman, Melanie Davies, Azhar Farooqi, David Kingdon, Ian Lawrence, Steve Longworth, Paul McNally and Tim Terry. The final responsibility for what follows is mine. Colour photographs are courtesy of Paul McNally.

I thank my wife and children for their good-natured tolerance of my absences in mind, if not in body. I dedicate this book to them with gratitude and love.

List of Abbreviations

4S, Scandinavian Simvastatin Survival Study
AAMI, Association for the Advancement of Medical Instrumentation Standard
ACAT, acyl coenzyme A cholesterol acyltransferase
ACE, angiotensin-converting enzyme
ACR, albumin:creatinine ratio
ADA, American Diabetes Association
AER, albumin excretion rate
ALLHAT, antihypertensive and lipid lowering to prevent heart attack trial
ARA, angiotensin-II receptor antagonists
ATHENS, Access to Higher Education via NISS Authentication System
BHF, British Heart Foundation
BHS, British Hypertension Society
BMI, body mass index
BNF, British National Formulary
CALM, candesartan and lisinopril microalbuminuria
CARE, cholesterol and recurrent events
CBT, Cognitive behaviour therapy
CCBs, calcium channel blockers
CETP, cholesteryl ester transfer protein
CHD, coronary heart disease
CK, creatine kinase
CRD, Centre for Reviews and Dissemination
CSMO, clinically significant macular oedema
CVD, cardiovascular disease
DARE, database of abstracts of reviews of effect
DCCB, dihydropyridine CCBs
DCCT, Diabetes Control and Complications Trial
DoH, Department of Health
DPP , Diabetes Prevention Program
DREAM, Diabetes Reduction Assessment with Ramipril and Rosiglitazone Medication
DVLA, Driver and Vehicle Licensing Agency
EBM, evidence-based medicine
emp, enzyme modification of porcine insulin
GI, glycaemic index
GLP-1, glucagon-like peptide-1
GMP, guanosine monophosphate
GP, general practitioner
GPRD, General Practice Research Database
HAZ, Health Action Zone
HbA1c, haemoglobin A1c
HDL, high-density lipoprotein
HDL-C, HDL cholesterol
HIV, human immunodeficiency virus
HONK, Hyperosmolar nonketotic hyperglycaemic coma
HOPE, Heart Outcomes Prevention Evaluation

HTA, health technology assessment
IDDM, insulin-dependent diabetes mellitus
IDF, International Diabetes Federation
IFG , impaired fasting glucose
IGT, impaired glucose tolerance
LDL, low-density lipoprotein
LDL-C, LDL cholesterol
LFT, liver function test
LIFE, Losartan Intervention for Endpoint Reduction in Hypertension
LIPID, Long-Term Intervention with Pravastatin in Ischaemic Disease
LVH, left ventricular hypertrophy
MI , myocardial infarction
MIMS, Monthly Index of Medical Specialities
MNT, medical nutritional therapy
MODY, maturity onset diabetes of the young
MRC, Medical Research Council
NeLH, National electronic Library of Health
NHS, National Health Service
NHS EED, NHS economic evaluation database
NICE National Institute of Clinical Excellence
NIDDM, non-insulin-dependent diabetes mellitus
NIH, American National Institute of Health
NPH, neutral protamine Hagedorn
NRT, nicotine replacement therapy
NSF, National Service Framework
OGTT, oral glucose tolerance test
PILs, patient information leaflets
PPAR-γ, peroxisome proliferator-activated receptor-gamma
PPRG, postprandial glucose regulator
prb, proinsulin synthesised by bacteria
pyr, precursor synthesised by yeast
QUIDS, Quality Indicators for Diabetes Services
RAPRIO, reassurance, advice, prescription, referral, investigations, observation
RCGP, Royal College of General Practitioners
RCTs, randomised controlled trials
SIGN, Scottish Intercollegiate Guidelines Network
SSRI, selective serotonin reuptake inhibitor
STOP-NIDDM, Study to Prevent NIDDM
T2ARDIS, Type 2 Diabetes: Accounting for a Major Resource Demand in Society in the UK
TG, triglyceride
TRIP, Turning Research into Practice
TZD, thiazolidinediones
VLCD, very low calorie diet
WHO, World Health Organisation
WOSCOPS, West of Scotland Coronary Prevention Study

CHAPTER ONE

Introduction: Why is Primary Care Important in the Management of Type 2 Diabetes Patients?

Diabetes mellitus is defined as a metabolic disease characterised by chronic hyperglycaemia. Its subgroup type 2 (see Chapter 2 for details of diagnosis and classification), previously known as noninsulin-dependent diabetes mellitus (NIDDM), accounts for the overwhelming majority of patients who have diabetes. Patients with diabetes can present in primary care with a wide range of problems, either as a direct manifestation of diabetes or with diabetes being a significant cause of the presentation. Although considerable expertise is available in secondary care, there are four good reasons why primary care should take a greater, or even leading, role in the delivery of care to patients with diabetes, and allow secondary care to concentrate on the more complex and challenging cases:

- The adverse impact of diabetes upon patients;
- The increasing prevalence of diabetes and demands upon secondary care;
- The importance of quality in the delivery of care to patients with diabetes;
- The suitability of primary care to manage chronic diseases.

Adverse Impact of Diabetes upon Patients

Patients with diabetes, especially type 2, are prone to a wide and devastating range of complications, predominately vascular. The United Kingdom Prospective Diabetes Study (UKPDS) showed, in a series of articles published in 1998, that many diabetic complications can be prevented or reduced by appropriate interventions,[1-3] many of which can be carried out in primary care. Compared with the general population, type 2 diabetics have a markedly greater risk of suffering myocardial infarction and stroke, particularly if additional vascular factors are present (as they often are). Diabetic care needs to include evidence-based aggressive interventions that reduce vascular risk in diabetics[4] (see Chapters 8 and 9), as well as optimal management of the disease itself.

Increasing Prevalence of Diabetes and Demands upon Secondary Care

The prevalence of type 2 diabetes continues to increase, particularly in certain subgroups such as Indo-Asians, and results in a greater incidence of vascular disease in these already high-risk individuals (see Chapter 3). This rising prevalence will lead inexorably to a greater clinical workload in health services and an increasing financial impact on various services. The progressive failure of overstretched hospital-based services to cope with these problems will result, inevitably, in primary care teams taking on an even greater proportion of diabetic care in the future. UK primary care studies show that the proportion of patients with diabetes (both types 1 and 2) who regularly attend hospital clinics for their diabetic care is low: 50% for inner city practices and 20–30% for suburban and rural practices.[5]

It is clear that effective, sustained and coordinated strategies to prevent or delay the onset of diabetes need to be implemented to counter this rise in its prevalence. This is discussed in greater detail in Chapter 3.

Importance of Quality in Delivering Care to Patients with Diabetes

In October 1989, government health departments and patients' organisations from across Europe, under the aegis of the World Health Organisation (WHO) and the International Diabetes Federation (IDF), agreed unanimously upon a series of recommendations for diabetes care to be implemented. Called the St Vincent Declaration, this set out goals and targets for improved and effective care.[6,7] Subsequent initiatives in the UK, some of which are discussed below, have built upon this landmark declaration.

A central aim of government health policy is improved quality of service to individual patients and to the whole population.[8] The term clinical governance refers to the range of activities needed to achieve this improved quality.[9] All health care professionals will be expected to become involved with a variety of initiatives, from national down to practice level, aimed at implementing clinical governance.[10] Recent and proposed changes to general practitioners' (GPs) contracts with the National Health Service (NHS) reflect the government's intention to support and reward improved quality of care in various areas, including diabetes.

Improved quality of care should be attainable in chronic diseases such as diabetes, based upon implementation of agreed and justified protocols in combination with audit to evaluate performance and guide future changes. Some diabetic patients do not have regular contact with their practice, and those who do attend can receive a variable standard of care.[11] Poor organisation can reduce the benefit diabetic patients could obtain from professionals' often-considerable knowledge and skills.

Several authoritative guidelines for the management of diabetes are now readily available:

1 The aim of the National Service Framework (NSF) for Diabetes is to 'make the best practice already offered in some places the norm' in a ten-year programme beginning in 2003. Publication was in two stages. The first stage, published in December 2001, lists 12 'standards' (*Table 1.1*), of which eight are relevant to type 2 diabetes management in primary care and define the areas of care that will need to be delivered by all involved agencies and health care professionals;[12] however, these standards are more aims than detailed recommendations for clinical practice as set out in the guidelines mentioned below. Text in this book that is specific to these standards is indicated by a symbol in the margin (as in the margin here), in which the

NSF X

number X changes according to the relevant standard. The second stage, published in January 2003 sets out a strategic framework on how the NHS, particularly at local level, will implement the NSF standards over a ten year programme (uncosted)[13]. The three main elements are:

- In the first year PCTs will be expected to put into place the basic organisation (setting up a diabetes network) and to begin to build capacity (baseline assessments, participation in comparative audits and workforce development).
- Within the first 3 years (2003–2006) the priority will be to achieve two specific targets: eye screening and the use of practice-based registers. By 2006, 80% of people with diabetes should be offered retinal screening, rising to 100% by the end of 2007. In primary care, practice-based registers should be updated so that patients with coronary heart disease (CHD) and diabetes continue to be managed in line with NSF standards.

Table 1.1. National Service Framework for diabetes standards and where they are discussed herein

Standard	Where discussed
1. *Prevention:* To reduce the number of people who develop type 2 diabetes	Chapter 3: prevention Chapter 7: dietary advice Chapter 12: exercise
2. *Diagnosis:* To ensure that people with diabetes are identified as early as possible	Chapter 2: diagnosis Chapter 4: screening
3. *Empowerment:* To ensure that people with diabetes are empowered to enhance their personal control over the day-to-day management of their diabetes in a way that enables them to experience the best quality of life	Chapter 5: organisation Chapter 7: monitoring, diet Chapter 12: education Chapter 14: information sources
4. *Clinical Care:* To maximise the quality of life of all people with diabetes and to reduce their risk of developing the long-term complications of diabetes	Chapter 5: organisation, recall Chapter 7: glycaemic control Chapter 9: cardiovascular risk Chapter 8: periodic review Chapter 13: audit
5. *Young People with Diabetes:* High-quality care	Type 1 diabetes – not in the scope of this book
6. *Young People with Diabetes:* Smooth transition from paediatric to adult services	Not in the scope of this book
7. *Diabetic Emergencies:* To minimise the impact on people with diabetes of the acute complications of diabetes	Chapter 10: metabolic and vascular emergencies Chapter 7: monitoring
8. *Hospital Admissions*	Not in the scope of this book
9. *Diabetes and Pregnancy*	Not in the scope of this book
10. *Detection and Management of Long-term Complications:* All patients with diabetes receive regular surveillance for the long-term complications of diabetes	Chapter 5: organisation Chapter 8: periodic review
11. *Detection and Management of Long-term Complications:* Implement and monitor agreed protocols of care so that all those who develop complications receive appropriate care	Chapter 8: periodic review Chapter 13: audit
12. *Detection and Management of Long-term Complications:* All those who require multi-agency support will receive integrated health and social care	Chapter 5: organisation Chapter 8: periodic review

By March 2006 the target is to ensure that these registers and systematic treatment regimens (including appropriate lifestyle advice) cover the majority of patients at high risk of CHD [particularly those with hypertension, diabetes and a body mass index (BMI) greater than 30].

- Over the ten years 2003–2006 the NHS will aim to reach all 12 NSF standards. The government expects that the 'overarching goal' of primary care trusts will be to provide tangible service improvements from 2003.

2 The National Institute of Clinical Excellence (NICE) was established in 1999 to provide guidance on new and existing technologies and to develop clinical guidelines and audit tools. NICE has already published its appraisals on the glitazones, anti-obesity drugs and insulin glargine, with likely future appraisals to include angiotensin-converting enzyme (ACE) inhibitors.

3 The National Clinical Guideline for type 2 diabetes consists of six inter-related guidelines, developed by a multi-professional, multi-agency collaboration with the support of NICE. These guidelines (with regular updating) aim to provide clinical practice recommendations (with the supporting evidence) for health care professionals in the following key areas:

- Foot care (prevention and management of foot problems), published in 2000 by the Royal College of General Practitioners.[14] An amended updating of this guideline is due to published by NICE in late 2003.
- Retinopathy (diabetic retinopathy: early management and screening), with a summary published in 2002 by NICE,[15] and the more detailed guidelines and supporting evidence published in 2001 by the Effective Clinical Practice Unit, University of Sheffield.[16]
- Renal care (renal disease: prevention and early management), with a summary published in 2002 by NICE,[17] again with more detailed guidelines and supporting evidence published in 2002 by the Effective Clinical Practice Unit, University of Sheffield.[18]
- Lipids management, with detailed guidelines and supporting evidence published in October 2002.[19]
- Blood pressure management, with detailed guidelines and supporting evidence published in October 2002.[20] Both the clinical guidelines for the management of blood lipids and blood pressure are summarised in a NICE document published in October 2002.[21]
- Blood glucose management, with a summary by NICE,[22] and more detailed guidelines and supporting evidence by the Effective Clinical Practice Unit, University of Sheffield,[23] both published in 2002.

These guidelines are discussed in detail later in this book. While it is not 'politically correct' to advise deviation from official guidance, this author believes that the NICE guidance has not always been set out clearly and that some of its recommendations are inconsistent with its own stated targets, other current authoritative guidance and the results of research (such as of the UKPDS). Professionals need to take on board this information, but ultimately they should not be afraid to exercise their best clinical judgement to act in their patients' best interests.

4 The Scottish Intercollegiate Guidelines Network (SIGN) published its own excellent authoritative guidelines in November 2001.[24]

5 The American Diabetes Association (ADA) publishes comprehensive and referenced clinical practice recommendations that are updated annually, available on its website.[25]

Implementing any guidance is likely to require extra resources, since our patients deserve nothing less than the vigorous and effective implementation of an appropriate agreed care package.

Suitability of Primary Care to Manage Chronic Diseases

Many health care professionals recognise now that, unlike acute diseases in which patients are usually passive recipients of medical care, successful chronic disease management requires the patient to be an active partner in the process.[26] This principle is the basis of patient empowerment, cited in NSF Standard 3 (*Table 1.1*). If the patients are regarded as the main managers of their chronic disease, with the professionals acting as both guide and coach, then better compliance and better outcomes are more likely. Primary care professionals are better placed to facilitate this than their colleagues in secondary care because:

- Primary care is more geared to focusing on the 'whole' patient and to addressing his or her agenda;
- Primary care is more accessible; and
- Patients may prefer the continuity of seeing their GP and practice nurse rather than a succession of junior hospital doctors in a busy hospital diabetic clinic.

Although intensive blood-glucose control increases therapy costs (drugs, monitoring, clinic visits), the UKPDS has argued these are offset largely by significantly reduced costs of complications, particularly if these result in hospital outpatient visits and/or admissions.[27]

Well-organised and highly motivated practices can provide both high-quality and cost-effective care for the majority of type 2 diabetic patients. Better management of chronic diseases can provide health care professionals with increased job satisfaction and with the opportunity to work as part of a multi-disciplinary practice team.

Key Messages of the Book

- The predominant damage to patients with type 2 diabetes is vascular.
- The core aims of the management of type 2 diabetes should be both the reduction of vascular risk and the improved well-being of patients.
- Collaboration between patients (achieving and maintaining an optimal lifestyle) and health care professionals (implementing agreed evidence-based interventions) is more likely to achieve these aims.
- Patients own their disease, and thus they are at the centre of goal setting and disease management.
- Health education is more about modifying attitudes than imparting information.
- The remorseless rise in the prevalence of type 2 diabetes will place increasing demands upon health services, especially primary care.
- Effective prevention strategies at all levels require immediate implementation with adequate resources to reduce the rising prevalence and impact of type 2 diabetes.

REFERENCES

1 UK Prospective Diabetes Study Group. Tight blood pressure control and risk of macro vascular and micro vascular complications in type 2 diabetes: UKPDS 38. *BMJ* 1998; 317: 703–712.

2 UK Prospective Diabetes Study Group. Intensive blood-glucose control with sulphonylureas or insulin compared with conventional treatment and risk of complications in patients with type 2 diabetes (UKPDS 33). *Lancet* 1998; 352: 837–853.

3 UK Prospective Diabetes Study Group. Effect of intensive blood-glucose control with metformin on complications in overweight patients with type 2 diabetes (UKPDS 34). *Lancet* 1998; 352: 854–865

4 Byrne CD, Wild SH. Diabetes care needs evidence-based interventions to reduce risk of vascular disease (Editorial). *BMJ* 2000; 320: 1554–1555.

5 Williams DRR. Health services for patients with diabetes in the 1990s. In: Jarrett RJ, Ed. *Diabetes Mellitus.* London: Croom Helm, 1986: 57–75.

6 WHO/IDF. Diabetes care and research in Europe: the St Vincent's Declaration. *Diabet Med* 1990; 7: 360.

7 Krans HMJ, Porta M, Keen H, Eds. *Diabetes Care and Research in Europe. The St Vincent Declaration action programme.* Implementation document. Copenhagen: World Health Organisation, Regional Office for Europe, 1992.

8 Department of Health. *A First Class Service.* London: Department of Health, 1998.

9 Department of Health. *Clinical Governance: quality in the new NHS.* Health Circular: HSC 1999/065. London: Department of Health, 1999.

10 Rosen R. Clinical governance in primary care: Improving quality in the changing world of primary care. *BMJ* 2000; 321: 551–554.

11 Audit Commission. *Testing Times: a review of diabetes services in England and Wales.* London: The Audit Commission, 2000.

12 Department of Health. *National Service Framework for Diabetes: Standards.* London: HMSO, 2001.

13 Department of Health. *National Service Framework for Diabetes: Delivery strategy.* London: HMSO, 2002.

14 Hutchinson A, McIntosh A, Feder G, *et al. Clinical Guidelines for Type 2 Diabetes: prevention and management of foot problems.* London: Royal College of General Practitioners, 2000.

15 NICE Guideline Development Group and Recommendations Panel. *Inherited Clinical Guideline E. Management of type 2 diabetes: retinopathy – screening and early management.* London: NHS National Institute for Clinical Excellence, 2002. Online: http://www.nice.org.uk

16 Hutchinson A, McIntosh A, Peters J, *et al. Clinical Guidelines for Type 2 Diabetes: diabetic retinopathy: early management and screening.* Sheffield: ScHARR, University of Sheffield, 2001. Online: http://www.shef.ac.uk/guidelines/

17 NICE Guideline Development Group and Recommendations Panel. *Inherited Clinical Guideline F. Management of type 2 diabetes: renal disease – prevention and early management.* London: NHS National Institute for Clinical Excellence, 2002. Online: http://www.nice.org.uk

18 McIntosh A, Hutchinson A, Marshall S, *et al. Clinical Guidelines and Evidence Review for Type 2 Diabetes: renal disease: prevention and early management.* Sheffield: ScHARR, University of Sheffield, 2002. Online: http://www.shef.ac.uk/guidelines

19 McIntosh A, Hutchinson A, Feder G, *et al. Clinical Guidelines and Evidence Review for Type 2 Diabetes. Lipids management.* Sheffield: ScHARR, University of Sheffield, 2002. Online: http://shef.ac.uk/guidelines

20 Hutchinson A, McIntosh A, Griffiths CJ, *et al. Clinical Guidelines and Evidence Review for Type 2 Diabetes. Blood pressure management.* Sheffield: ScHARR, University of Sheffield, 2002. Online: http://shef.ac.uk/guidelines

21 NICE Guideline Development Group and Recommendations Panel. *Inherited Clinical Guideline H. Management of type 2 diabetes: management of blood pressure and blood lipids.* London: NHS National Institute for Clinical Excellence, 2002. Online: http://www.nice.org.uk

22 NICE Guideline Development Group and Recommendations Panel. *Inherited Clinical Guideline G. Management of type 2 diabetes: management of blood glucose.* London: NHS National Institute for Clinical Excellence, 2002. Online: http://www.nice.org.uk

23 McIntosh A, Hutchinson A, Home PD, *et al. Clinical Guidelines for Type 2 Diabetes: blood glucose management.* Sheffield: ScHARR, University of Sheffield, 2002. Online: http://www.shef.ac.uk/guidelines/

24 Scottish Intercollegiate Guidelines Network. *Clinical Guidelines: management of diabetes.* Edinburgh: Scottish Intercollegiate Guidelines Network. Online: http://www.sign.ac.uk/

25 American Diabetes Association. *Clinical Practice Recommendations.* Online: http://www.diabetes.org.

26 Holman H, Lorig K. Patients as partners in managing chronic disease. *BMJ* 2000; 320: 526–527.

27 Gray A, Raikou M, McGuire A, *et al.* Cost effectiveness of an intensive blood glucose control policy in patients with type 2 diabetes: economic analysis alongside randomised control trial (UKPDS 41). *BMJ* 2000; 320: 1373–1378.

CHAPTER TWO

What is Type 2 Diabetes Mellitus?

Definition of Diabetes Mellitus

Diabetes mellitus is a group of metabolic diseases characterised and diagnosed by a chronic elevation of blood glucose (hyperglycaemia) that results from defects in insulin secretion, insulin action or both. This may be accompanied by a variety of disturbances of carbohydrate, protein and fat metabolism. The impact of clinical manifestations may depend upon the underlying cause(s) of the diabetes, the degree of deficit of insulin action, coexisting conditions and the extent of diabetic tissue damage.

Classification of Diabetes Mellitus

WHO proposed a classification of diabetes in 1980, modified in 1985,[1] and this was adopted internationally. The American Diabetes Association's Expert Committee on the Diagnosis and Classification of Diabetes Mellitus, in parallel with WHO, re-examined the diagnostic criteria and classification and recommending certain modifications in 1997, which were subsequently agreed by WHO.[2,3] Type 1 and type 2 diabetes (*Table 2.1*) replace the old categories of insulin-dependent diabetes mellitus (IDDM) and NIDDM. The older classification was based upon treatment (but many NIDDM patients are on insulin) and does not indicate the underlying problem.[4]

Types 1 and 2 diabetes have significant differences, as shown in *Table 2.2*.

Disease Processes of Type 2 Diabetes Mellitus

Type 2 diabetes is a heterogeneous disease,[6] but its chronic hyperglycaemia results from diverse and progressive disease processes that cause both:

- Defects in the ability of pancreatic beta cells to secrete insulin (beta cell dysfunction); and
- Defects in the ability of insulin to inhibit hepatic glucose production and to promote glucose utilisation (insulin resistance).

In type 2 diabetes, both of these defects coexist and both can be caused by a plethora of genetic or environmental factors. Most commonly, type 2 diabetes appears to be inherited as a polygenic trait, with environmental factors also involved, often at a very young age (as discussed below and in Chapter 3).

Secretion of insulin, in response to rising blood glucose levels, occurs in *two* phases in healthy individuals:

Table 2.1. 1997–1998 ADA and WHO classification of diabetes mellitus

Type 1 (beta-cell destruction, usually leading to absolute insulin deficiency)

Autoimmune
Idiopathic

Type 2 (may range from predominately insulin resistance with relative insulin deficiency to a predominately secretory defect with or without insulin resistance)

Other specific types

Genetic defects of beta-cell function
Genetic defects in insulin action
Diseases of the exocrine pancreas
Endocrinopathies
Drug- or chemical-induced
Infections
Uncommon forms of immune-mediated diabetes
Other genetic syndromes sometimes associated with diabetes

Gestational diabetes mellitus (includes gestational impaired glucose tolerance)

1. The first (early acute) phase consists of a rapid rise in insulin immediately after an increase in blood glucose levels. This insulin is thought to originate from a small pre-formed reserve pool of insulin stored within the beta cells.
2. The second (late) phase response consists of a more gradual rise in insulin levels. The on-going biosynthesis of newly formed insulin in this phase occurs during the time that blood glucose levels are elevated.

Early in type 2 diabetes, beta cells begin to lose their initial response of increased insulin secretion ('first phase'). Sustained hyperglycaemia may cause a further reduction in beta cell function by 'glucose toxicity'. With progression of the disease, the loss of first-phase secretion leads to exaggerated early post-prandial hyperglycaemia, exaggerated late ('second-phase') insulin secretion and late post-meal hypoglycaemia. Insulin secretory pulses become abnormal under basal conditions. Worryingly, the loss of first-phase insulin secretion, which leads to post-prandial glucose 'spikes', is associated with an increased risk of cardiovascular disease.

In insulin resistance, insulin is unable to produce its usual effects at concentrations that are effective in normal individuals. Its onset precedes the development of type 2 diabetes and may arise from a variety of genetic mutations (so it may be partly inherited). It is thought that the reduced action of insulin is linked closely with the cardiovascular risk factors, such as obesity, that are part of the insulin resistance syndrome.[7]

Malnutrition *in utero* and during early infancy may be associated with an increased risk of developing type 2 diabetes later in life (the 'thrifty phenotype' hypothesis) by affecting both beta cell function and insulin resistance. Regular physical exercise, when undertaken consistently from childhood, can protect against type 2 diabetes by improving insulin sensitivity.

Table 2.2. Comparison of the characteristics of types 1 and 2 diabetes mellitus[5]

Characteristic	Type 1	Type 2
Age at onset	Usually <30 years	Most often >30 years, but note recent trends
Associated obesity	No	Yes
Propensity to ketoacidosis, requiring insulin to control	Yes	No
Presence at diagnosis of classic symptoms of hyperglycaemia	Yes, often severe	May be absent If present, often moderate
Endogenous insulin secretion	Very low to undetectable	Variable, but low relative to plasma glucose levels
Insulin resistance	Not present	Yes, but variable
Twin concurrence	<50%	>90%
Associated with specific HLA-D antigens	Yes	No
Islet cell antibodies at diagnosis	Yes	No
Islet pathology	Insulitis, selective loss of most beta cells	Smaller, normal-looking islets Amyloid deposits common
Associated risks for micro- and macrovascular disease	Yes	Yes
Hyperglycaemia responds to oral agents	No	Yes, initially in many patients

Biochemistry of diabetic complications

In addition to being a strong risk factor for the development of CHD, type 2 diabetes is associated with progressive and specific damage to the small vessels of certain target organs, primarily the retina, the renal glomerulus and the peripheral nervous system. These tissues are freely permeable to glucose. Poor glycaemic control renders such tissues more vulnerable to insult, which starts insidiously and leads on to failure of the related major systems. The clinical consequences of diabetic microvascular disease are visual impairment, chronic renal failure and neuropathic foot ulceration (discussed in Chapter 8). Animal studies suggest the following hypotheses for tissue damage that results from chronic exposure to high glucose concentrations:

1 Increased activity of the *polyol pathway* leads ultimately to depletion of *myo*-inositol and impairment of Na^+, K^+-adenosinetriphosphatase (ATPase) activity, implicated in the pathogenesis of diabetic neuropathy.

2 Accumulation of diacylglycerol activates protein kinase C-b in endothelial cells, which alters the vascular permeability and increases basement membrane synthesis. This may contribute to the development of new vessels in the retina (proliferative retinopathy).

3 *Nonenzyme glycation* is the attachment of glucose to the amino groups of proteins at a rate proportional to the mean glucose concentration (the basis of glycated haemoglobin assay to measure medium-term glycaemic control). This long-term alteration of proteins appears to contribute to tissue damage.

Criteria and Methods for the Diagnosis of Diabetes Mellitus

NSF
2

Concepts involved in making a diagnosis

In theory, the diagnosis of diabetes mellitus should be straightforward: the blood glucose level is either above or below the diagnostic threshold. However, the reality is not so simple in type 2 diabetes! Consensus must be reached as to what level of plasma glucose should be set as the diagnostic threshold (*criteria*) and which diagnostic test(s) to use (*methods*). Making the correct diagnosis reliably in an asymptomatic patient (half of type 2 patients are so at diagnosis) poses a challenge.

Current criteria and methods

Both criteria and methods of diagnosis have been revised over the years. The current recommendations, adopted in the UK from 1st June 2000, are based on the WHO consultative document produced in 1998.[3] The following criteria are for diagnosis only and are *not* treatment criteria or goals of therapy:

1 Plasma glucose level in a patient with classic symptoms (e.g., thirst, polyuria, lethargy, blurred vision and weight loss) *on a single occasion*:
   • Fasting level of 7.0mmol/l (126mg/dl) or greater; or
   • Random level of 11.1mmol/l (200mg/dl) or greater; or
   • A 2 hour post 75g glucose load of 11.1mmol/l or greater, from an oral glucose tolerance test (OGTT; see below).
2 Plasma glucose levels in an asymptomatic patient, based upon *two abnormal results on separate days*:
   • Fasting level of 7.0mmol/l or greater, or
   • Random level of 11.1mmol/l or greater, or
   • A 2 hour post 75g glucose load of 11.1mmol/l or greater, from an OGTT.

Although the OGTT is the 'gold standard', it should not normally be regarded as a first-line investigation in general practice, unless the fasting or random plasma glucose results fail to resolve uncertainty over the diagnosis. This is most likely in patients whose fasting plasma glucose levels fall into the 'impaired fasting glucose' range (see below), especially if they are thought to be at high risk of developing either diabetes or vascular disease. These individuals probably need to have an OGTT performed.

The presence of glycosuria, an abnormal finger-prick blood glucose or an elevated glycated haemoglobin is suggestive, but does not satisfy the diagnostic criteria for diabetes.

Rationale for diagnostic criteria and methods

Determining the optimal diagnostic level of hyperglycaemia depends upon balancing the medical, social and economic costs of making a diagnosis in someone not truly at substantial risk of the adverse effects of diabetes with the costs of failing to diagnose someone who is at substantial risk. The distribution of plasma glucose concentrations is a continuum, but there is an approximate threshold that separates those subjects who are at a substantially increased risk for some adverse outcomes caused by diabetes (e.g., microvascular complications) from those who are not.[8]

Although WHO and other bodies have adopted ADA's diagnostic criteria proposed in 1997,[2] they have differed over the optimal method of diagnosis. WHO has always preferred OGTT. The DECODE Study Group found that the 2 hour post-load plasma glucose levels were more accurate than fasting plasma glucose levels in identifying individuals at an increased risk of death associated with hyperglycaemia.[9] The drawback of ADA's strong preference for fasting plasma glucose levels is that 'normal' results carry the risk of missing some individuals with diabetes, especially among the elderly and in some ethnic groups (see discussion below). This is not altogether surprising, since the early defect in the natural history of beta cell dysfunction is the reduction of first-phase insulin release, associated with 2 hour post-load hyperglycaemia, while second-phase insulin release may stay normal initially, as reflected in a normal fasting plasma glucose level.

Oral glucose tolerance test
Standard protocol
After 3 or more days with a daily carbohydrate intake of at least 150g, the OGTT is performed in the morning after an overnight fast of 8 to 14 hours (during which plain water may be drunk). Once fasting has been confirmed, a venous blood sample is taken and a drink that contains the equivalent of 75g of glucose (e.g. Lucozade 388ml) is consumed over not more than 5 minutes. The subject should be seated, not smoke and take no unusual exercise during the test period. A second venous blood sample is taken exactly 2 hours after the start of the glucose drink. Both samples should be sent to an accredited laboratory for estimation of plasma glucose. Interpretation of the results of the OGTT test is given in *Table 2.3*.

Impaired glucose tolerance and impaired fasting glucose
These terms are not interchangeable and do not define identical groups of individuals. Impaired glucose tolerance (IGT) refers to a glucose metabolic state that is intermediate between normal glucose homeostasis and diabetes mellitus. Strictly speaking, the term IGT should only refer to a plasma glucose level of between 7.8 and 11.0mmol/l at 2 hours after a 75g glucose load. Therefore, patients should be labelled as having IGT only after an OGTT, whereas impaired

Table 2.3. Interpretation of the OGTT[8]

Based on plasma venous glucose	Fasting	2 hours post 75g glucose load
Diabetes mellitus	7.0mmol/l or greater	11.1mmol/l or greater
Impaired glucose tolerance	–	7.8–11.0mmol/l
Impaired fasting glucose	6.1–6.9mmol/l	–
Normal glucose homeostasis	6.0mmol/l or less	7.7mmol/l or less

fasting glucose (IFG) refers only to a fasting plasma glucose level of between 6.1 and 6.9mmol/l. As suggested above, some patients, particularly elderly or Indo-Asians, can have IFG, but fulfil the diagnostic criteria for diabetes because their 2 hour post 75g load plasma glucose level is 11.1mmol/l or greater. Thus, patients with IFG can have either diabetes or IGT or normal glucose homeostasis (based upon the 2 hour result). This has major implications for screening (see Chapter 4), because a fasting plasma glucose level below the diagnostic threshold for diabetes does not exclude current diabetes reliably.

Individuals with IGT are at increased risk of developing macrovascular disease, consistent with the findings of the DECODE study. Also, 15% of individuals with IGT will become type 2 diabetics within 10 years. Thus, it is logical to regard IGT as a risk factor rather than as a clinical entity, particularly as many individuals with IGT are asymptomatic and have normal plasma glucose levels in their daily lives. Some evidence suggests that the most cost-effective interventions to prevent or delay the onset of diabetes should target individuals with IGT, followed by high-risk groups (see the discussion on prevention in Chapter 3).

Key Points in this Chapter

- Type 2 diabetes is characterised by a chronic elevation of blood glucose, which results from defects in insulin secretion, insulin action (also known as insulin resistance) or both.

- The criterion for diagnosis is a plasma glucose level either randomly of 11.1mmol/l or greater or fasting of 7.0mmol/l or greater or 2 hours post 75g glucose load of 11.1mmol/l or greater from an OGTT – on a single occasion if symptomatic or on two separate occasions if asymptomatic.

- Impaired glucose tolerance is a significant predictor of diabetes and macrovascular disease.

REFERENCES

1 WHO Study Group on Diabetes Mellitus. *Diabetes Mellitus.* Technical Report Series No. 727. Geneva: WHO, 1985.

2 The Expert Committee on the Diagnosis and Classification of Diabetes Mellitus. Report of the Expert Committee on the diagnosis and classification of diabetes mellitus. *Diabetes Care* 1997; 20: 1183–1197.

3 Alberti KGMM, Zimmet PZ for the WHO Consultation. Definition, diagnosis and classification of diabetes mellitus and its complications. Part 1: Diagnosis and classification of diabetes mellitus. Provisional report of a WHO Consultation. *Diabet Med* 1998; 15: 539–553.

4 Wroe CD. Conference Report from the 57th Annual Meeting and Scientific Sessions of the ADA. *Practical Diabetes Int* 1997; 14: 142.

5 Beers MH, Berkow R, Eds. *The Merck Manual of Diagnosis and Therapy,* 17th Edn. Whitehouse Station: Merck Research Laboratories, 1999.

6 Kumar S, Barnett AH. Causes of non-insulin dependent diabetes mellitus. *Diabet Med* 25: 6–9.

7 Reaven GM. Insulin resistance in human disease. *Diabetes* 1988; 37: 1595–1607.

8 The Expert Committee on the Diagnosis and Classification of Diabetes Mellitus. Report of the Expert Committee on the diagnosis and classification of diabetes mellitus. *Diabetes Care* 2003; 26(Suppl. 1): S5–S20.

9 DECODE Study Group on behalf of the European Diabetes Epidemiology Study Group. Glucose tolerance and mortality: Comparison of WHO and American Diabetes Association diagnostic criteria. *Lancet* 1999; 354: 617–621.

CHAPTER THREE

Impact of Type 2 Diabetes

Epidemiology of Type 2 Diabetes

Current prevalence

The precise overall prevalence of diabetes in the UK at the beginning of the twenty-first century is not known, as no large-scale community studies have been carried out recently using a standardised glucose challenge. However, a number of studies over the past 10 years have attempted to estimate prevalence.

In 1996 researchers in Tayside, Scotland, found the prevalence for all diabetes to be 1.93% (with 89.2% of these being type 2) using electronic record linkage of multiple data sources.[1] If extrapolated to the estimated total UK population in 1996, at least 1,060,000 people had type 2 disease. A report from NICE estimated that about 2.4% of the adult population have been diagnosed with diabetes mellitus and that about 80% of these (800,000 individuals in England and Wales) have type 2 disease.[2] Researchers using data from the General Practice Research Database (GPRD) calculated the prevalence of diagnosed diabetes (all types) in 1998 to be 1,150,000 in England and Wales (age-standardised prevalence of 2.23 per 100 males and 1.64 per 100 females). This study did not formally calculate the prevalence of type 2 diabetes, but, as three-quarters of this population were diet controlled or on oral hypoglycaemic medication[3] and many type 2 diabetics are treated with insulin, the vast majority of the diabetics in this study were type 2.

All these prevalence figures are likely to be underestimates, because many type 2 patients are asymptomatic *and* the individuals and/or their health care professional may not always recognise the symptoms of hyperglycaemia.

Future prevalence

The prevalence of type 2 diabetes looks set to continue to increase rapidly in the future. It has been estimated that the worldwide prevalence of type 2 diabetes will more than double from 98.9 million in 1994 to 215 million by 2010.[4] This extrapolates to two million patients in the UK diagnosed by 2010. The study cited above, using the GPRD, predicted that the prevalence of diabetes in England and Wales would rise to 1,660,000 by 2023, especially in an increasingly ageing population.

Factors that affect the prevalence of type 2 diabetes

Ethnic origin

The prevalence is particularly high in populations that have changed from a traditional to a modern life-style, such as migrant Afro-Caribbeans and Indo-Asians in the UK. Indo-Asians are not a homogeneous group, with the greatest prevalence being in Pakistanis, then in Bangladeshis and finally in Indians.

Age

The peak age of onset of type 2 diabetes is 60 years. Most subjects are diagnosed after 40 years of age. However, a younger age of onset is now occurring more frequently, especially in certain high-prevalence ethnic groups, such as Indo-Asians and Afro-Caribbeans, and in individuals with very adverse factors for insulin resistance (i.e. obesity, sedentary lifestyle and unhealthy diet). Maturity onset diabetes of the young (MODY) syndromes, which are genetic defects of beta cell function, are classified separately from type 2 diabetes.

Obesity

Obesity, especially truncal, is associated closely with type 2 diabetes. The risk increases as the BMI rises. Obesity is more likely to occur with the wrong diet and lack of physical exercise. Eating less and exercising more are at the core of programmes to delay or prevent the onset of type 2 diabetes. Recently, four cases of type 2 diabetes in very obese (BMI greater than 35kg/m^2) white adolescents were reported,[5] and widely publicised in the lay press. This frightening phenomenon, likely to become more common in the future, increases the priority to resource and to implement wide-ranging effective health education programmes aimed at preventing type 2 diabetes.

Deprivation

Deprivation is associated with a higher prevalence in both sexes aged 35 to 74 years,[3] although it is unclear whether this is independent of the above factors.

Diabetic Control, Mortality and Complications

Overall, 5-year mortality in type 2 diabetes increases two- to three-fold and age-adjusted life expectancy is reduced by 5–10 years compared to the general population,[6] with 58% of all mortality in type 2 diabetes related to cardiovascular disease alone.[7]

Both the Department of Health (DoH)[8] and the St Vincent Declaration[9] identified the role of health care professionals in improving diabetic care and, in particular, of setting targets for the reduction of complications. The adverse effects of sustained hyperglycaemia and poor management on mortality and morbidity in type 2 diabetes have been studied extensively. In type 1 patients, tight glycaemic control[10] and early appropriate intervention have been shown to reduce the impact of diabetic complications. The UKPDS has now identified poor glycaemic control among the risk factors for coronary artery disease in patients with type 2 diabetes.[11] The UKPDS also demonstrated that very good glycaemic control significantly reduced the risk of both microvascular complications (e.g., retinopathy, nephropathy) and macrovascular disease (e.g., CHD, major stroke) in patients with type 2 diabetes.[12,13]

As many type 2 patients at diagnosis have evidence of complications, particularly vascular, and/or the presence of cardiovascular risk factors, early diagnosis (including targeted screening, as discussed in Chapter 4) and high-quality management can improve their future well-being.

Financial Impact of Type 2 Diabetes

While the rising prevalence of diabetes will increase patient suffering and health care professionals' workload, it will also cause headaches for Chancellors of the Exchequer and whoever else has responsibility for financing health care. Currently, 4–5% of the total health care expenditure in the NHS is for the care of people with diabetes mellitus, including the cost of dealing with complications.[8] It has been predicted that this could rise to 10% of total NHS expenditure by 2011.[14] Diabetic complications are a major major contributor these high costs. The estimated total annual cost of treating diabetic foot problems alone in the UK was £13 million in 1994.[15]

The project Type 2 Diabetes: Accounting for a Major Resource Demand in Society in the UK (T2ARDIS) looked at the financial impact of type 2 diabetes and presented its results at the British Diabetic Association's (now Diabetes UK) Professional Conference in March 2000.[16] T2ARDIS calculated that the average annual direct cost to the country of treatment for each person with type 2 diabetes in 2000 to be £2151, comprising:

- £1738 (81%) to the NHS, the total annual cost being £2 billion, which is 4.7% of total NHS expenditure, and of this hospitalisation consumes more than 40%.
- £285 (13%) borne by the private individual.
- £129 (6%) allocated to the social services. Over 75% of social services' costs for people with type 2 diabetes are associated with residential and nursing care.

T2ARDIS also showed that the presence of both microvascular and macrovascular complications in an individual increases NHS costs five-fold, personal expenditure three-fold and social services' costs four-fold.

Any measures that reduce the medical impact of diabetes (by prevention, earlier detection or improved care to reduce complications) should also reduce its financial impact.

Prevention of Type 2 Diabetes Mellitus

In view of the above, what can be done to prevent type 2 diabetes? The predicted rise in prevalence makes the need to consider and to implement effective preventive strategies all the greater. Prevention or delay of the onset of diabetes reduces cardiovascular risk (see Chapter 9).

NSF
1
3

Certain factors, such as age, ethnic origin and family history, are beyond an individual's control. However, many individuals who develop type 2 diabetes have a less than optimal lifestyle, over which they do have control. Factors associated with increased cardiovascular risk and greater insulin resistance are already present in British children, particularly of Indo-Asian origin.[17] Eating a healthier diet (see Chapter 7) and undertaking increased and appropriate exercise (see Chapter 8) reduces insulin resistance.

Published studies of prevention of diabetes

Published studies demonstrate that diabetes in high-risk individuals can be prevented either by improving lifestyle (by weight reduction, dietary modification and increased physical activity) or by medication. These warrant a brief discussion.

Modifying lifestyle

The Da Qing IGT and Diabetes Study (China), published in 1997, followed up 577 individuals with IGT over 6 years, showed a reduction by at least one-third of the incidence of new diabetes with either diet or exercise interventions or both.[18]

The Finnish Diabetes Prevention Study Group, published in 2001, followed up 522 overweight individuals with IGT over a mean of 3.2 years, and compared 'individualised' counselling aimed at reducing weight, modifying diet and increasing physical activity against controls. The cumulative incidence of new diabetes was reduced by 58% in the intervention group compared to the control group, or one case of diabetes was prevented for every 22 overweight individuals with impaired glucose tolerance 'treated' for 1 year.[19]

The Diabetes Prevention Program (DPP) in the USA, published in 2002, followed up 3234 'high-risk' subjects over a mean of 2.8 years, and compared three arms: standard lifestyle recommendations plus placebo, standard lifestyle recommendations plus the biguanide drug metformin, and an intensive programme of lifestyle modification (16 lessons covering diet, exercise and behaviour modification). The reduction in incidence of new cases of diabetes was 31% in the metformin group (treat 41.7 subjects for 1 year to prevent one new case) and 58% in the intensive programme group (treat 20.7 subjects for 1 year to prevent one new case).[20]

It must not be forgotten that to apply any of the above programmes on a sustained basis to a large population will require considerable resources.

Medication

Effective prevention of diabetes using medication is a potentially massive market for pharmaceutical companies. Even if proved effective, the colossal financial costs of treating large populations with some of these drugs may be prohibitive. Four agents show promise in the prevention of new cases of diabetes:

- An incidental finding in the Heart Outcomes Prevention Evaluation (HOPE) trial was the lower rate of new diagnosis of diabetes in vascular high-risk patients aged over 55 years treated with the ACE inhibitor ramipril.[21] As a result, a large prospective trial is underway to study individuals with impaired glucose tolerance, the Diabetes Reduction Assessment with Ramipril and Rosiglitazone Medication (DREAM) study.
- The DPP (cited above) demonstrated a reduction in incidence of type 2 diabetes in high-risk subjects who used metformin, but lifestyle changes were even more effective as prevention.[20]
- In the multicentre Losartan Intervention for Endpoint Reduction in Hypertension (LIFE) study, which looked at cardiovascular morbidity and mortality in 9193 patients with essential hypertension and left ventricular hypertrophy and compared treatment using the angiotensin-receptor antagonist losartan with atenolol, new onset diabetes was less common in the losartan-treated group.[22]
- In another multicentre randomised trial, Study to Prevent NIDDM (STOP-NIDDM), conversion of impaired glucose tolerance into type 2 diabetes was less in patients treated with the alpha-glucosidase inhibitor acarbose than with placebo. However, 31% of the patients allocated to the acarbose group discontinued treatment early.[23] Unfortunately, the use of acarbose is limited by frequent gastrointestinal side effects (see Chapter 8).

The findings of the HOPE and LIFE studies support evidence from previous studies that inhibition of the renin–angiotensin system may improve glucose tolerance. The LIFE study authors suggested an effect on insulin resistance, but other hypotheses suggest an increased insulin secretory response, either by inducing a raised pancreatic islet blood flow to secure a better early insulin response[24] or as a result of the higher serum potassium levels associated with ACE-inhibitor use augmenting insulin secretion[25] Further research is needed.

Prevention issues that need to be resolved

There is no simple magical solution to this problem. Societies and their health services will need to look at many measures at levels that range from individuals to whole populations.

Successful health education requires collaboration and a unity of purpose, from appropriate government policies down to practice level. Health professionals have an important role, but are not the only players here. Government policy is reflected in Chapter 6 of the NSF Diabetes' Strategy, which refers to national initiatives and best-practice models that tackle diet, physical activity and smoking cessation, particularly in schools and/or deprived areas.[26]

The huge demand placed upon finite resources (financial and human) is one of the main barriers to applying and sustaining successfully any of the above interventions to a large population. The practical compromise may be to give priority to proved interventions in those individuals most likely to benefit.

Attempts to change an individual's behaviour raise the potential dilemmas that surround patient empowerment. The concept is laudable and may promote effective disease management in many cases, but individuals have the right to make choices that ultimately may cause them harm. Lifestyles are largely the result of choices made by individuals. Any intervention to alter these must respect each individual's right to make decisions and must assess each individual's willingness to change (the trans-theoretical model of change and techniques to change motivation are discussed in Chapter 12). Another challenge for health professionals and organisations is to develop clear and equitable policies in response to patient demands for available interventions that may lack full clinical justification or affordability within a limited budget.

Key Points in this Chapter

- About 2.4% of the adult population have been diagnosed with diabetes mellitus and about 80% of these (800,000 individuals in England and Wales) have type 2 disease, but these prevalence figures are likely to be underestimates. The prevalence is set to rise, with a prediction of 2,000,000 type 2 diabetics in the UK by 2010.

- Ethnicity (especially Indo-Asian), age and obesity are associated with increased prevalence.

- Five-year mortality in type 2 diabetes increases two- to three-fold and age-adjusted life expectancy is reduced by 5–10 years compared to the general population, with 58% of all mortality in type 2 patients caused by cardiovascular disease alone. Poor glycaemic control increases risk.

- Currently, 4–5% of the total health care expenditure in the NHS is for the care of people with diabetes mellitus, predicted to rise to 10% by 2011. Diabetic complications are a major cause of these high costs. T2ARDIS calculated that the average annual direct cost to the country of treatment for each person with type 2 diabetes is £2151.

- Factors associated with increased cardiovascular risk and greater insulin resistance are already present in British children, particularly those of Indo-Asian origin. Individuals can reduce their insulin resistance by eating a healthier diet and by undertaking increased and appropriate exercise.

REFERENCES

1 Morris AD, Boyle DI, MacAlpine R, *et al.* The diabetes audit and research in Tayside Scotland (DARTS) study: electronic record linkage to create a diabetes register. *BMJ* 1997; 315: 524–528.

2 National Institute for Clinical Excellence. *Guidance on Rosiglitazone for Type 2 Diabetes Mellitus.* London: Department of Health, 2000. Online: http://www.nice.org.uk

3 Newnham A, Ryan R, Khunti K, *et al.* Prevalence of diagnosed diabetes mellitus in general practice in England and Wales, 1994 to 1998. In National Statistics, *Health Statistics Quarterly*, Vol. 14. London: HMSO, 2002: 5–13. Online: http://www.statistics.gov.uk

4 Amos AF, McCarty DJ, Zimmet P. The rising global burden of diabetes and its complications: estimates and projections to the year 2010. *Diabet Med* 1997; 14: S7-S85.

5 Drake AJ, Smith A, Betts PR, *et al.* Type 2 diabetes in obese white children. *Arch Dis Child* 2002; 86: 207–208.

6 Panzram G. Mortality and survival in Type 2 (non-insulin dependent) diabetes mellitus. *Diabetologia* 1987; 30: 123–131.

7 Davies MJ, Burden AC, Burden ML. Screening for type 2: increasing evidence that it is necessary. Part 1: Should it be done? *Practical Diabetes Int* 1997; 14: 162–164.

8 Department of Health. *Health of the Nation.* London: HMSO, 1991.

9 WHO/IDF. Diabetes care and research in Europe: the St Vincent's Declaration. *Diabet Med* 1990; 7: 360.

10 The Diabetes Control and Complications Research Group. The effect of intensive treatment of diabetes on the development and progression of long-term complications in insulin-dependent diabetes mellitus. *N Engl J Med* 1993; 329: 977–986.

11 Turner RC, Millns H, Neil HAW, *et al.* for the United Kingdom Prospective Diabetes Study Group. Risk factors for coronary artery disease in non-insulin-dependent diabetes mellitus: United Kingdom prospective diabetes study (UKPDS: 23). *BMJ* 1998; 316: 823–828.

12 UK Prospective Diabetes Study Group. Intensive blood-glucose control with sulphonylureas or insulin compared with conventional treatment and risk of complications in patients with type 2 diabetes (UKPDS 33). *Lancet* 1998; 352: 837–853.

13 Stratton IM, Adler AI, Neil HAW, *et al.* Association of glycaemia with macrovascular and microvascular complications of type 2 diabetes (UKPDS 35): prospective observational study. *BMJ* 2000; 321: 405–412.

14 Boulton A. Non-insulin dependent diabetes needs more attention. *BMJ* 1996; 313: 510.

15 Williams DRR. The size of the problem; epidemiological and economic aspects of foot problems in diabetes. In: Boulton AJM, Conner H, Cavanagh PR, Eds. *The Foot in Diabetes,* 2nd Edn. Chichester: John Wiley and Sons, 1994: 15–24.

16 British Diabetic Association, King's Fund, Economists Advisory Group and SmithKline Beecham Pharmaceuticals UK, 2000. *T2ARDIS: Implications for Seamless Care Provision in Type 2 Diabetes in the UK.* Data presented at the Diabetes UK Professional Conference, 2000.

17 Whincup PH, Gilg JA, Papacosta O, *et al.* Early evidence of ethnic differences in cardiovascular risk: cross-sectional comparison of British South Asian and white children. *BMJ* 2002; 324: 635–638.

18 Pan XR, Li GW, Hu YH, *et al.* Effects of diet and exercise in preventing NIDDM in people with impaired glucose tolerance: the Da Qing IGT and Diabetes Study. *Diabetes Care* 1997; 20: 537–544.

19 Tuomilehto J, Lindstorm J, Eriksson JG, *et al.* for the Finnish Diabetes Prevention Study Group. Prevention of type 2 diabetes mellitus by changes in lifestyle among subjects with impaired glucose tolerance. *N Engl J Med* 2001; 333: 1343–1350.

20 Diabetes Prevention Program Research Group. Reduction in the incidence of type 2 diabetes with lifestyle intervention or metformin. *N Engl J Med* 2002; 346: 393–403.

21 Yusuf S, Gerstein H, Hoogwerf B, *et al.* (for the HOPE Study Investigators). Ramipril and the development of diabetes. *JAMA* 2001; 286: 1882–1885.

22 Dählof B, Devereux RB, Kjeldsen SE, *et al.* for the LIFE study group. Cardiovascular morbidity and mortality in the losartan intervention for endpoint reduction in hypertension study (LIFE): a randomised trial against atenolol. *Lancet* 2002; 359: 995–1003.

23 Chiasson J-L, Josse RG, Gomis R, *et al.* for The STOP-NIDDM Trial Research Group. Acarbose for prevention of type 2 diabetes: the STOP-NIDDM randomised trial. *Lancet* 2002; 359: 2072–2077.

24 Carlsson PO, Berne C, Jansson L. Angiotensin II and the endocrine pancreas: effects on islet blood flow and insulin secretion in rats. *Diabetologica* 1998; 41: 127–133.

25 Santoro D, Natali A, Palombo C, *et al.* Effects of chronic angiotensin converting enzyme inhibition on glucose tolerance and insulin sensitivity in essential hypertension. *Hypertension* 1992; 20: 181–191.

26 Department of Health. *National Service Framework for Diabetes: Delivery strategy.* London: HMSO, 2002.

CHAPTER FOUR

Should we be Screening for Type 2 Diabetes Mellitus?

General Points and Definitions

In addition to making a diagnosis and carrying out effective and appropriate management, health care systems need to consider whether an active search for new cases of diabetes is worthwhile. Diagnostic testing and screening are distinctly different processes. When an individual exhibits clinical features of a condition, diagnostic testing using standard criteria is performed. This does not represent screening. Screening aims to identify asymptomatic individuals likely to have that condition, followed by appropriate diagnostic tests.

How Strong is the Case for Screening for Type 2 Diabetes?

The benefits of screening should be evaluated against recognised criteria.[1,2] These are summarised as:

1 *The prevalence of the disease in the population to be screened must be sufficient to make mass screening practical.* As discussed in Chapter 3, the prevalence of type 2 diabetes in the total UK population is estimated to be at least 1.9% and is rising. This prevalence is greater with increasing age, particularly ethnicity (Indo-Asians) and/or the presence of one or more other risk factors (hypertension, obesity, family history of diabetes).[3] Targeted screening of these groups would require less resource and produce a higher yield (hence, be more practical) than screening the whole population.

2 *The disease must be clearly defined to allow an accurate diagnosis.* There have been clear diagnostic criteria for type 2 diabetes since 1985,[4] last updated in 2000.

3 *There should be evidence that the disease is undiagnosed in a significant proportion of individuals, so that a prompt early diagnosis is not inevitable in most of these cases.* There is good evidence that most type 2 diabetes patients have had their disease at least 4–7 years prior to clinical diagnosis.[5] Diabetes UK recently launched a publicity campaign to increase public awareness of this asymptomatic phase. Complications are evident in many patients at diagnosis.

4 *Early diagnosis of the disease must result in improved outcomes, including disease treatment and reduced impact of complications.* It is worrying that at least one-third of patients with type 2 diabetes have at least one complication present when diagnosed.[6] However, type 2 diabetes patients identified by screening have:
- A significant cluster of cardiovascular risk factors, which can be improved by early intervention;[7]
- A lower prevalence of microvascular complications at diagnosis;[6] and
- A lower risk of death than in known type 2 diabetes patients after 4 years in a UK study.[8]

Furthermore, patients found to have IGT may benefit from interventions to reduce both their risk of becoming diabetic in the future and of their existing propensity to develop cardiovascular disease. Ultimately, the practice must be able to offer high-quality, appropriate and effective care on a consistent basis to newly diagnosed diabetics.

5 *The screening test(s) used must be readily available and must have an acceptable specificity, sensitivity and predictive value in the population to be screened.* Reliable blood-glucose estimation is readily available by sending samples to an accredited local chemical pathology laboratory. All three ways of diagnosing diabetes listed in Chapter 2 have a high sensitivity (i.e., the likelihood of a positive result in patients with disease) and positive predictive value, because they define the disease, which is a lifelong diagnosis. However, a negative OGTT has a higher specificity (i.e., the likelihood of a negative result in patients without disease) than a negative fasting or random plasma glucose, because a proportion of diabetics can be missed by the latter two screening tests. The predictive value of a negative result is not entirely conclusive, since currently nondiabetic individuals, particularly from higher risk groups, may become diabetic in the future. A result that demonstrates IGT, although negative for diabetes, does predict an increased risk of developing diabetes later.

6 *The screening test(s) used must be acceptable to individuals being screened, and not cause significant adverse effects.* Venepuncture is invasive, but is regarded as low risk when performed by a competent person. Most individuals would probably find it acceptable.

7 Other criteria are:
- Case finding and treatment must be cost-effective, in relation to health expenditure as a whole;
- Facilities and resources must be available to treat newly diagnosed cases;
- Screening must be a systematic on-going process and not merely an isolated one-time effort.

Primary care is well placed to develop the accurate population and disease registers required to identify at-risk subjects, and to undertake regularly both recall and screening tests, provided that adequate systems are in place and maintained (Chapter 5). However, any systematic and sustained programme requires sufficient additional resources for screening, diagnostic tests and treatment, and these must be balanced against other demands made upon the practice.

Practical Issues in Screening for Type 2 Diabetes

Consideration of the above shows that any practice seeking to screen a population for type 2 diabetes needs to consider four practical questions:

1 Who to screen?
2 How to screen?
3 How often to screen?
4 Is the practice able to provide high-quality care to newly diagnosed diabetics without detriment to other patients?

Additional evidence is required to resolve fully the uncertainties that surround the first three questions, a point recognised by the Diabetes NSF. The UK National Screening Committee has requested additional research into screening, and it plans to report to the DoH in 2005.[9] A practice's decisions need to be based upon what is most feasible, both logistically and clinically.

Who to screen?

Evidence of target organ damage (eyes, kidneys and feet) should prompt the clinician to consider whether the patient is diabetic. The case for screening the whole population for type 2 diabetes is not yet proved. In addition to a lower yield of new cases, whole-population screening requires considerable staff time (calculated as 1 hour per week for a year to screen 620 patients in that period[3]). However, a recent screening programme that recruited well elderly Americans demonstrated that the presence of certain factors (age, gender, ethnicity, raised BMI, greater waist:hip ratio, hypertension) increased the yield to as much as one new case of diabetes diagnosed for every six individuals screened.[10]

Until the DoH guidance appears, the current consensus is for a targeted screening approach that concentrates on the following 'high-risk' groups:

- Members of high-risk ethnic groups, that is Indo-Asians and Afro-Caribbeans, over 60 years of age;
- Individuals with a first-degree relative with diabetes;
- Individuals with recurrent or major sepsis;
- The obese (20% or more above ideal weight);
- Individuals with peripheral skin breakdown (e.g., ulcers);
- Individuals with autoimmune endocrinopathies (e.g., primary hypothyroidism) or organ-specific disorders (e.g., polycystic ovary disease);
- Women with a history of gestational diabetes or who have delivered a baby that weighs more than 9 pounds (4kg);
- Individuals with CHD (logical in light of the high risk of this in type 2 diabetics);
- Individuals that had IGT on previous testing.

It is sensible for the organiser of the screening programme to create a register of these 'high-risk' individuals to facilitate recall.

Which screening method to use?

The rationale for the different diagnostic methods is discussed in Chapter 2. However, the logistics and greater resource demands of the OGTT render it unsuitable to be undertaken as the first-line test on a large scale in primary care. The less sensitive and specific fasting plasma glucose test may be the optimal compromise as the initial screening test. However, as noted in Chapter 2, fasting plasma glucose has a reduced specificity because many individuals, particularly Indo-Asians, with a nondiabetic fasting level will have a diabetic level at 2 hours post glucose load. If the fasting blood glucose is just below the diagnostic threshold (from 6.0–6.9mmol/l, i.e., impaired fasting glucose) or if the patient is at high risk of developing diabetes, then diagnostic certainty requires performing either a 2 hour post glucose load blood glucose or an OGTT. Neither urine testing (simple, quick and cheap) nor glycated haemoglobin are suitable because they do not fulfil the diagnostic criteria for diabetes.

How often to screen?

Diabetes UK recommends (but the supporting evidence is not cast-iron) that screening should not be performed more often than every 5 years in subjects with no risk factors, and no more often than every 3 years in those with one risk factor. A UK study suggests that screening using post-prandial urinalysis for glycosuria should be repeated at 2- or 3-year intervals,[11] but it is not clear whether this applies to the other screening methods.

Practices should consider what interventions to undertake between screening in those individuals identified as negative for diabetes, but at higher risk. Although additional evidence is required, common sense suggests that to minimise cardiac risk factors by health education (smoking, diet, exercise) and by intervention (blood pressure control, serum lipids) is appropriate.

Is the practice able to provide high-quality care to newly diagnosed diabetics without detriment to other patients?

While recognising the strong arguments in favour of targeted screening for diabetes, a practice should not forget that:

- Screening will require additional resources, particularly of staff time.
- The newly diagnosed diabetic patient should receive high-quality, appropriate and effective care on a consistent basis.
- The delivery of care to other patients with existing diabetes and/or other significant problems must be maintained and not suffer when additional tasks are taken on.

Key Points in this Chapter

- Many issues related to screening for type 2 diabetes remain unresolved and await official guidance.
- Early detection of the disease reduces its impact.
- Depending upon the availability of resources, regular screening of high-risk individuals, using fasting plasma glucose (with an OGTT in selected individuals), is feasible in primary care.

REFERENCES

1 Davies MJ, Burden AC, Burden ML. Screening for type 2: increasing evidence that it is necessary. Part 1: Should it be done? *Practical Diabetes Int* 1997; 14: 162–164.

2 Expert Committee on the Diagnosis and Classification of Diabetes Mellitus. Position Statement: screening for diabetes. *Diabetes Care* 2003; 26(Suppl. 1): S21–S24.

3 Lawrence JM, Bennett P, Young A, *et al.* Screening for diabetes in general practice: cross-sectional population study. *BMJ* 2001; 323: 548–551.

4 WHO Study Group on Diabetes Mellitus. *Diabetes Mellitus.* Technical Report Series No. 727. Geneva: WHO, 1985.

5 Harris MI, Klein R, Welborn TA, *et al.* Onset of type 2 occurs at least 4–7 years before clinical diagnosis. *Diabetes Care* 1992; 15: 815–819.

6 UK Diabetes Information Audit and Benchmarking Service (UKDIABS). London: Diabetes UK, 2000.

7 Davies MJ, Grenfell A, Day JL. Clinical characteristics and follow-up of subjects with non-insulin-dependent diabetes mellitus diagnosed by screening. *Practical Diabetes Int* 1996; 13: S42.

8 Croxson SCM, Price DE, Burden ML, *et al.* The mortality of elderly people with diabetes. *Diabet Med* 1994; 11: 250–252.

9 Department of Health. *National Service Framework for Diabetes: Standards.* London: HMSO, 2001.

10 Franse LV, Bari MD, Shorr RI *et al.* Type 2 diabetes in older well-functioning people: who is undiagnosed? Data from the Health, Aging and Body Composition Study. *Diabetes Care* 2001; 24: 2065–2070.

11 Davies MJ, Day JL. Screening for non-insulin dependent diabetes mellitus: how often should it be performed? *J Med Screen* 1994; 1: 78–81.

CHAPTER FIVE

Organising the Delivery of Optimal Care

Aims and Values

NSF
3
4
10
11
12

It is common for organisations to publish some type of formal statement of their aims (or goals or objectives) and of the values (or means or methods) that govern their behaviour. If the area of activity is complex and the individuals who work in an organisation have diverse roles, it is beneficial for all to be aware of that organisation's core aims and values. Knowledge of or referral to explicit sensible aims and values can improve decision-making both by organisations (about how to deliver care) and by patients and professionals (about how to best manage each patient's diabetes). The two stages of the Diabetes NSF set out not just what optimal care should be,[1] but how it might be delivered.[2] However, those charged with delivering care need to recognise that the targets likely to be set for various metabolic and vascular variables (discussed in detail in Chapter 8) may not be achievable in all cases and may involve polypharmacy, which risks both a reduction in compliance and an increase in the adverse effects.

For the whole practice population with type 2 diabetes

The delivery of high-quality care to type 2 diabetic patients in a primary care setting requires that their needs are identified clearly and correctly (such as through audit) and that the available resources are used optimally to address these needs. This is most likely in a practice:

• That is *motivated* to provide the highest standards of care;
• Whose members are *skilled*, and receive regular and appropriate training; and
• That is *well organised*.

Table 5.1 summarises suggested organisational aims for a practice diabetic population.

Table 5.1. Delivery of care to the practice diabetic population

Suggested aims

Be efficient and effective based upon clear evidence

Address the needs of both individual patients and the whole practice population

Be committed to equal access by and equal responsiveness to people from all socioeconomic, ethnic and cultural backgrounds

Integrate all involved members of the primary health care team (professional and support)

Work seamlessly with secondary care and relevant outside agencies

Ensure appropriate quality control with regular monitoring (such as audit)

Table 5.2. Suggested aims for the outcomes of care for individuals with diabetes

Ensure the earliest possible detection of the disease

Abolish symptoms of the disease

Achieve optimal blood glucose control, avoiding hypoglycaemia

Prevent and provide early treatment of any potential complications

Reduce the risk and impact of cardiovascular disease

Enable the patients to play the fullest possible role in the management of their disease, by providing suitable education and psychological support

For the individual patient with type 2 diabetes

The best possible outcomes are more likely if the aims of the organisation that delivers the care (as in *Table 5.1*) respect and complement the goals chosen by each individual diabetic patient. As discussed below, patients are the main managers of their disease and all professionals need to respect and support this. Diabetic patients who understand their disease, which is a chronic condition that is almost always a lifelong diagnosis, are more likely to share the same aims as the caring professional. *Table 5.2* summarises a professional's perspective of suitable aims for the care of individual patients with diabetes.

Components of optimal organisation within primary care

Achieving the above-stated aims does not occur spontaneously. Effective delivery of care to diabetics has relied traditionally upon the three Rs of chronic disease management: Registration, Recall and regular Review. However, recently published evidence indicates that 'multifaceted' interventions (such as individualised goal-setting with patients and suitable education) improve the performance of both the practitioners and the organisation, with better outcome measurements of such parameters as blood pressure and glycated haemoglobin.[3,4] A successful 'recipe' for diabetic care needs the appropriate ingredients, as shown in *Table 5.3*.

Table 5.3. Overview of the likely necessary components in an organisation that delivers diabetic care successfully

Active participation of diabetic patients in their care

Access to committed trained professionals with a suitable range of skills

Effective administrative structures and processes

Optimal information management

Adequate physical premises and equipment

Access to suitable information for patients and professionals

Active participation of diabetic patients in their care

As stated above, patients with diabetes should be regarded as the main managers of their chronic disease, with the professional acting as both guide and coach. This is more likely if professionals respect their patients' autonomy.

Attention to the following guiding principles should enhance this autonomy and the quality of diabetic care delivered:

• It must be remembered that type 2 diabetes is a progressive disease that requires regular and staged changes in therapy. Patients must not be made to feel guilty or at fault when these changes occur.

• Treatment plans should be 'negotiated' and should attempt to incorporate each patient's own chosen goals. Other issues and concerns in a patient's life may affect the priority given to these diabetes-related goals.

• Interventions should aim to promote and maintain improved self-care behaviour[5] and to maximise freedom and flexibility in the patient's life.

• Where possible, patients should be encouraged to adjust their treatment and be supported in this. Patients will need to know the actual values and the significance of any tests. This requires the professional to identify and address each patient's educational needs. If patients are allowed to make decisions, then they should be allowed, without stigmatisation, to make mistakes from which each patient and the professional can learn. Remember, patients own their disease.

• The professional should aim to earn and maintain each patient's respect. Solid evidence, where available, should support any guidance given.

• Both the patients and the professional should remember that a balance needs to be struck between keeping things as simple as possible and recognising that diabetes is not a simple disease.

• In respecting each patient's autonomy and empowerment, the professional must remember that patients have the right to make choices that may ultimately cause them harm.

Primary health care team personnel

The following principles should enhance the effectiveness of the team members who deliver diabetic care:

• The practice team (i.e., doctors, nurses and administrative staff) needs to be committed and enthusiastic about delivering diabetic care. Otherwise, it will be drudgery and done abysmally. The active leadership of a GP or a practice nurse with a particular interest in diabetes is likely to provide the necessary driving force within the team.

• The members of the practice involved in the scheme require sufficient knowledge and skills to carry out their tasks. Training needs may be identified by a variety of methods, including appraisals, audit, questionnaires and patient feedback. Training may be obtained from a variety of sources, such as attendance at specific courses, observation of specialist colleagues or clinics, distance learning, self-directed reading (see Chapter 14) or in-house. Regular updates of knowledge and skills are necessary, as in any medical field.

• Nonmedical members of the team can and should play a leading role. With adequate training and safeguards, nurses should be able to prescribe changes in therapy according to an agreed protocol; this enables a prompt and more effective response to problems and a greater likelihood that the individual patient's goals will be achieved.

• Good working relationships with others involved in diabetic care outside the practice, both in health and in other services (e.g., social), will facilitate each patient's access to and a more seamless movement between the available agencies that best address each particular need. Cultivation of local primary care trusts or groups to take an increasing interest in the practices' activities may attract both practical support and additional resources.

- All team members must be committed to ensuring equitable access and care to patients of all ethnic and cultural backgrounds. Developing good relationships with social and religious organisations within the local community should facilitate this.

Chapter 6 of the Diabetes NSF *Delivery Strategy*[2] outlines issues that relate to workforce planning and development. Although directed more at a district level, the document and its references may be relevant to how individual practices might manage their own personnel.

Administrative structures and processes

Administrative structures and processes require the following:

1 Accurate up-to-date *diabetic register* for recall, management and audit (one of the Diabetes NSF priority targets, see Chapter 1), with a named person responsible for it. Most registers are computerised. All members of the practice must be encouraged to notify the register when made aware of a newly diagnosed or registered diabetic. Practices also need to consider setting up a parallel register of those at higher risk of developing diabetes, for recall to be screened regularly.

2 An *evidenced-based protocol* to cover all the key areas of diabetic care within the practice, such as diagnosis, screening, acute problems, periodic review and formulary. The NSF standards[1] and NICE-sponsored clinical guidelines for type 2 diabetes[6-10] should form the basis of the protocol, but there are several other sources for ideas, such as locally produced guidelines, Diabetes UK recommendations,[11] the Royal College of General Practitioners (RCGP)[12], SIGN[13] and the ADA.[14] It is crucial that every participating member of the team understands and agrees with the protocol once it is produced. Regular audit and reviews of medical literature should result in periodic revisions to the protocol.

3 An effective *call and recall system* should be in place. Administrative and clinical members need to agree the precise protocol (including standard recall letters) for contacting diabetic patients when and after their periodic review is due.

4 *Contact details* (telephone and fax numbers, and e-mail addresses) of outside professionals, such as diabetes specialist nurses, podiatrists and hospital diabetic, renal and eye clinics, should be available to the team members who deliver care.

5 The *framework for undertaking* both full and interim *diabetic reviews* should be agreed. Adequate time must be set aside within the framework to carry out properly the activities set out in the diabetic protocol. Where practices organise specific sessions for diabetic care, such as in dedicated diabetes mini-clinics, there is no difference between this and hospital clinics in terms of process and outcome.[15] There are various models for how time is organised:

- Mini-clinics, which are regular sessions set aside for diabetes care by the primary health care team, with regular participation from other professionals, such as hospital doctors, diabetes specialist nurses, dieticians and podiatrists. The author believes that, by organising for the relevant blood tests (as indicated in the periodic review's protocol) to be taken a few weeks prior to the mini-clinic, better management is more likely because all the relevant information is available at the time of review.

- Individual appointments with sufficient time for a review to be made available in the course of a session, but studies have shown that hospital and mini-clinics deliver superior care.

- The community care model is being developed, wherein a block of appointments for more than one practice can take place on a single site. These clinics can also bring in outside professionals.

Whichever model is chosen depends upon the practice team's assessment of its diabetic population's needs and the practice's capabilities. A possible model for the flow of patients through a practice is shown in *Figure 5.1*.

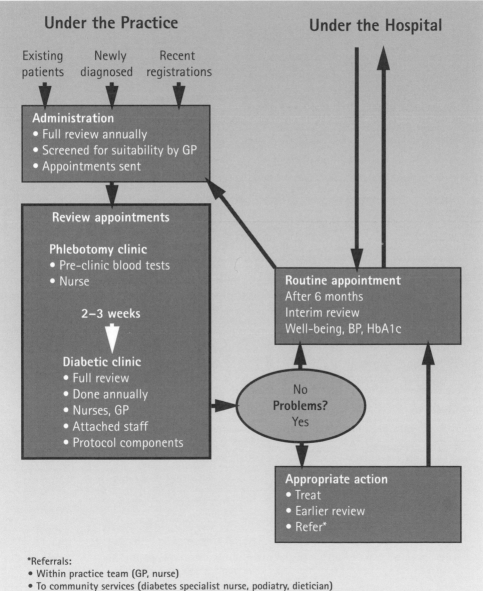

Figure 5.1 Flow of diabetic patients through the practice (HbA1c, haemoglobin A1c)

6   The structure for undertaking interim reviews and other important interventions varies considerably, depending upon the practice's appointments system and available resources. However, practices may wish to look imaginatively at *alternatives to the standard appointment* in the surgery or a home visit, particularly in lifestyle interventions (see Chapter 12). Examples include telephone prompting, group sessions, electronic and written educational packages, and the involvement of professionals from outside the primary health care team.

7   The practice should be capable of and willing to undertake regular *audit* and to implement changes (see Chapter 13), as cited in the NSF and very much at the centre of NHS clinical governance.

8   The practice must ensure that *adequate resources* are available for the relevant team members to carry out the entire range of tasks required to provide a high-quality service, without detriment to other professional activities.

Information management

Optimal information management is an essential ingredient in achieving improved quality in any area of health care. Strategic planning in this area needs to look at the content (what is recorded) and the system (how information is handled). Practices may wish to refer to the DoH's documents *Diabetes Information Strategy*[16] and *Information for Health.*[17]

Content

The data recorded by each practice are determined by clinical, administrative and medicolegal requirements. Any data recorded must have a clear purpose and should not be only 'for information's sake'. The components of the periodic review described in Chapter 8 and the areas for audit listed in Chapter 13 could provide the basis for the data that practices may wish to record. Precise definitions of all recorded data need to be agreed and understood by all users. All current UK electronic systems use Read Codes (details available from the NHS Information Agency[18]), although it is possible that Read Codes may be replaced in the near future by an internationally used American medical coding system. Where multiple codes are available for single or similar terms, practices should agree, where possible, a unique code for each item of data to be recorded.

System design

Whether the information system is electronic or manual, its design must address:

- Recording of data;
- Data storage;
- Data retrieval.

Recording of data

Data recording needs to be accurate, efficient and to facilitate retrieval.

In a manual system, diabetic data from regular reviews and other contacts can be recorded either in chronological sequence in the main notes or on a separate diabetic summary card. If the diabetic review data are recorded in the main notes, a stamp with the essential data headings can save writing and act as a useful prompt.

In an electronic system, diabetic data are best recorded onto agreed specific templates (like stamps in manual records), which facilitates data collection and its future accessibility. A clear decision is needed as to whether the clinician or a member of the support team actually enters the diabetic data onto the computer.

Irrespective of whether the system is manual or electronic, it is necessary to devise a practical and accurate system for recording data produced from outside the practice (e.g., hospital clinics) onto the practice database.

Data storage

Manual patient records should be identified easily as belonging to diabetic patients (i.e., tagged with a recognised coded sticker). Electronic records should be stored automatically on the practice computer's hard drive, but regular back-up stored off site is required in the event of crashes or disasters (e.g., fire).

Many patients and professionals support the creation of patient-held records to facilitate patient self-management and communication between different centres of care. However, it is necessary that all involved professionals have continuous access to the data. Electronic systems should minimise the time and effort devoted to duplicate data entry onto the practice database.

Data retrieval

With the increasing use of audit for administrative (e.g., contracts) and clinical purposes, the speed and accuracy of retrieving data for analysis on an electronic system is seen to far outweigh the initial extra effort of typical clinicians typing in their own data. A substantial proportion of receptionists' time is spent pulling and filing often-unwieldy sets of notes in a manual system, from which the accessibility of information is limited.

The storage and retrieval of patient data must respect all the relevant legal requirements, in particular the Data Protection Acts. This is a real minefield and any practice is well advised to have in place clear policies and suitable training for all involved staff.

Physical premises and equipment

Practices that carry out diabetic care have a need for the following (which may have 'resource implications'):

- Adequate space, including access to a darkened room for retinal screening, by whatever method (ophthalmoscope, slit-lamp or retinal camera).
- For clinical examination, to include a sphygmomanometer (with standard and large cuffs), an ophthalmoscope, mydriatic drops (tropicamide 0.5% and 1.0%), weighing scales, height measure, BMI chart, cotton wool, patella hammer, tuning fork (128Hz), sterile needles, 10g (5.07) monofilaments or Neurotips (if available), Snellen chart for visual acuity hung at the correct distance, and pinhole for correction of refractive errors.
- For testing, to include laboratory sample equipment (needles, syringes, blood and urine sample bottles, sharps container, disposable gloves and swabs), urine test strips (for protein, glucose and ketones), blood glucose meter and appropriate test strips (check with the local diabetic specialist nurse as to the favourite and ensure proper quality control) and finger pricking devices. Machines are now available for near-patient testing of glycated haemoglobin and other parameters, such as lipids and electrolytes. A practice's decision to acquire such equipment will be influenced by what it needs, the resource implications (costs, staff time) and the machine's reliability and accuracy (glycated haemoglobin assays should satisfy rigorous standardisation criteria that are difficult to achieve outside laboratories).

- For therapeutic indications, to include glucose for OGTT, and access to insulin and glucagon.
- For recording and management, to include, if electronic, a networked computer terminal with access to a printer for prescriptions and health education literature, and, if manual, the medical records and suitable stationery.

Patient information

Patient information includes:

- Educational materials (leaflets, posters and videos) should be available, if required, in appropriate languages for non-English speaking patients.
- Information on local services, including optician, dietician, podiatrist and social services.
- Links with patient-participation groups, either at practice level or at district level (such as Diabetes UK), are useful in providing further information and support.
- Lists of useful websites for patients with access to the internet (see Chapter 14).

Mary MacKinnon's book covers comprehensively all aspects of diabetes care in primary care, with much detail about all of the organisational issues.[19]

Delivering High-quality Care to Elderly Type 2 Diabetics

Type 2 diabetes in the elderly poses major clinical and logistical problems. Not only is the prevalence higher than in a younger population, but also these individuals are very likely to have significant macrovascular and microvascular disease. Furthermore, with increasing age, more will be house-bound or live in some form of residential or nursing home, and they are more likely than their nondiabetic contemporaries to request out-of-hours calls and to need acute hospital admission.[20] Staff in homes or other carers can feel isolated and, with numerous other demands upon their time, will not invariably monitor diabetic control and other problems to the highest possible standard.

There is no single simple solution to these problems. Practices will need to organise the provision of diabetic care at home for some individuals, in collaboration with other professionals, such as diabetes specialist nurses, podiatrists and opticians, and with the carer(s). Additional time and resources are likely to be required. It is crucial that the protocols are appropriate (not too complex or inflexible) and agreed by all those involved. Carers may require education and other support from the practice team. Optimal metabolic control is most likely if one motivated knowledgeable person is responsible.

Key Points in this Chapter

- Patients with diabetes should be regarded as the main managers of their chronic disease, with the professionals acting as both guide and coach.
- The delivery of high-quality care to type 2 diabetic patients in primary care is most likely in motivated, skilled and organised practices.
- The aims of diabetic care for each individual should be to:
  - ensure the earliest possible detection of the disease;

- abolish symptoms of the disease;
- achieve optimal blood glucose control, to avoid hypoglycaemia;
- prevent and provide early treatment of any potential complications;
- reduce the risk and impact of cardiovascular disease; and
- enable patients to play the fullest possible role in the management of their disease, by providing suitable education and psychological support.
- The components of optimal organisation include:
  - active participation of diabetic patients in their care;
  - access to committed trained professionals with a suitable range of skills;
  - effective administrative structures and processes;
  - optimal information management;
  - adequate physical premises and equipment;
  - access to suitable information for patients and professionals.

REFERENCES

1   Department of Health. *National Service Framework for Diabetes: Standards.* London: HMSO, 2001.
2   Department of Health. *National Service Framework for Diabetes: Delivery strategy.* London: HMSO, 2003.
3   Olivarus N de F, Beck-Nielsen H, Andreasen AH, *et al.* Randomised controlled trial of structured personal care of type 2 diabetes mellitus. *BMJ* 2001; 323: 970–975.
4   Renders CM, Valk GD, Griffin SJ, *et al.* Interventions to improve the management of diabetes mellitus in primary care, outpatient and community settings. *Cochrane Database Systematic Reviews* 2001; 1: CD001481.
5   Wolpert HA, Anderson BJ. Management of diabetes: Are doctors framing the benefits from the wrong perspective? *BMJ* 2001; 323: 994–996.
6   Hutchinson A, McIntosh A, Feder G, *et al. Clinical Guidelines for Type 2 diabetes: prevention and management of foot problems.* London: Royal College of General Practitioners, 2000.
7   NICE Guideline Development Group and Recommendations Panel. *Inherited Clinical Guideline E. Management of type 2 diabetes: retinopathy – screening and early management.* London: NHS National Institute for Clinical Excellence, 2002. Online: http://www.nice.org.uk
8   NICE Guideline Development Group and Recommendations Panel. *Inherited Clinical Guideline F. Management of type 2 diabetes: renal disease – prevention and early management.* London: NHS National Institute for Clinical Excellence, 2002. Online: http://www.nice.org.uk
9   Hutchinson A, McIntosh A, Peters J, *et al. Clinical Guidelines for Type 2 Diabetes: diabetic retinopathy: early management and screening.* Sheffield: ScHARR, University of Sheffield, 2001. Online:

http://www.shef.ac.uk/guidelines/
10 McIntosh A, Hutchinson A, Home PD, *et al. Clinical Guidelines for Type 2 Diabetes: blood glucose management.* Sheffield: ScHARR, University of Sheffield, 2002. Online: http://www.shef.ac.uk/guidelines/
11 Diabetes UK. *Recommendations for the Management of Diabetes in Primary Care.* 3rd Edn. London: Diabetes UK, 2000.
12 Royal College of General Practitioners. *Guidelines for the Care of Patients with Diabetes.* London: Royal College of General Practitioners, 1993.
13 Scottish Intercollegiate Guidelines Network. *Clinical Guidelines: management of diabetes.* Edinburgh: Scottish Intercollegiate Guidelines Network. Online: http://www.sign.ac.uk/
14 American Diabetes Association. *Clinical Practice Recommendations.* Online: http://www.diabetes.org.
15 Williams DRR. Health services for patients with diabetes in the 1990s. In: Jarrett RJ, Ed. *Diabetes Mellitus.* London: Croom Helm, 1986: 57–75.
16 Department of Health. *Diabetes Information Strategy.* London: Department of Health. 2003. Online: http://www.doh.gov.uk/ipu/strategy/nsf/dis.pdf.
17 Department of Health. *Information for Health.* London: Department of Health. 1998, updated 1999. Online: http://www.doh.gov.uk/ipu/strategy/index.htm.
18 NHS Information Agency. Online: http://www.nhsia.nhs.uk.
19 MacKinnon M. *Providing Diabetes Care in General Practice: A Practical Guide for the Primary Care Team,* 4th Edn. London: Class Publishing, 2002.
20 Tattersall R, Page S. Managing diabetes in residential and nursing homes. *BMJ* 1998; 316: 89.

CHAPTER SIX

The Newly Diagnosed Patient

Essential Questions to be Addressed at the Initial Contact

When the diagnosis of diabetes is made, three questions need to be answered by the clinician by the end of that initial consultation:

1 Is the patient severely ill?
2 Can this patient be managed in a primary care setting?
3 What treatment is required to correct blood glucose?

Is the patient severely ill?

If yes, an intercurrent illness is more likely to be the cause than type 2 diabetes, and the patient will require urgent admission to hospital, irrespective of the blood glucose level.

Can this patient be managed in a primary care setting?

Type 2 patients with treatable complications (i.e., major foot problems, renal failure and retinopathy) should be referred promptly to the appropriate hospital outpatient department. However, it is likely that the practice team will become involved in the subsequent management of these problems and of the diabetes.

What treatment is required to correct the blood glucose level?

Correction of elevated blood glucose begins at diagnosis. Using the 'step-up' recommendations outlined in *Table 7.3*, the initial choice of diet alone, oral hypoglycaemic agents or insulin is based upon the following:

- Current blood glucose level;
- Presence or absence of ketones in the urine;
- Presence of hyperglycaemic symptoms, such as polydipsia and polyuria;
- Patient's weight;
- Patient's general well-being, hepatic and renal function.

Required actions are outlined in *Table 6.1*.

Important Areas to Address from Diagnosis

At or soon after diagnosis, three further areas will require attention:

1 Involving the patient in the self-management of his or her disease;
2 Minimising cardiovascular risk (see Chapters 8 and 9);
3 Carrying out essential administrative tasks.

Table 6.1. Initial treatment of raised blood glucose in type 2 diabetes*

Evaluation	Action
Ketonuria present	Start insulin (step 4*)
Blood glucose >15mmol/l Hyperglycaemic symptoms present No ketonuria	Start oral hypoglycaemic agent (step 2*): metformin if obese; secretagogue if not obese
Blood glucose <15mmol/l No hyperglycaemic symptoms No ketonuria	Trial of diet (step 1*)

*Please refer also to *Table 7.3* and Chapter 7.

Involving the patient in self-management

From the first consultation, health care professionals need to educate patients about their condition, and allow the patients to make informed choices, wherever possible, about their management.

Minimising cardiovascular risk

An early assessment of overall vascular risk, followed by interventions to reduce or eliminate treatable risk factors, such as blood pressure, smoking and lipid profile, should be an integral part of the management of type 2 diabetes.

Immediate administrative tasks

The urgency of addressing these needs depends upon the patient's circumstances and clinical status (*Table 6.2*).

Early Assessment and Management

Remembering the aims of diabetic care stated in Chapter 5, the newly diagnosed type 2 patient requires an early full assessment to detect diabetic complications and cardiovascular risk factors, to identify any specific needs and to tailor management to these findings. This can be done either in the next available diabetic clinic session (if held regularly) or over a series of appointments. The components of the full periodic review (discussed in Chapter 8) are the basis of this assessment, which does need to be more comprehensive to establish a baseline. Additional information gathering may be indicated by the clinical situation. The structure of this assessment involves history, examination, investigations and administrative tasks (see *Table 6.2* and Chapter 8), and will enable the planning and implementation of the patient's optimal management. Success is more likely if the patient understands and agrees with the aims and methods. The familiar acronym RAPRIO (reassurance, advice, prescription, referral, investigations, observation) provides a useful framework to organise management:

- Reassurance:
  1 Be positive about the benefits of care.
  2 Address any fears or anxieties that the patients may have.

Table 6.2. Assessment of a newly diagnosed type 2 diabetic patient

History

Symptoms related to hyperglycaemia (i.e. thirst, polyuria, weight loss, tiredness)

Symptoms that may be related to diabetic complications: visual disturbance, angina, foot problems, sensory disturbances, diarrhoea, infections (balanitis, candidiasis) and male impotence

History and treatment of any other conditions

Life style (i.e., smoking, alcohol consumption, exercise, diet, other substance use)

Family history of diabetes and/or vascular disease

Social circumstances (e.g., occupation, others at home, cultural factors, health beliefs)

Mental status (e.g., cognitive function, affect – including any features of depression)

Examination

Height and weight to give BMI (kg/m^2)

Blood pressure: sitting and standing

Feet

Eyes: visual acuity, lens, fundus via dilated pupils

Oral examination

Thyroid palpation

Cardiac examination and peripheral pulses

Abdominal examination (e.g., for hepatomegaly an arterial bruits)

Neurological examination (e.g.,for neuropathy)

Investigations

Urinary glucose, protein and ketones. Send urine to microbiology laboratory to exclude infection if protein is detected. If screening for microalbuminuria, send first morning urine specimen to laboratory for albumin: creatinine ratio

Serum biochemistry: urea and electrolytes, possibly liver function

Serum total cholesterol, lipoprotein fractions and triglycerides

Thyroid function tests

Administrative tasks

Add to diabetic and annual influenza immunisation registers

Invite for pneumococcal immunisation if never administered before or for repeat immunisation either if with another immuno-comprising problem (see BNF) or if over 64 years of age and had previous immunisation more than 5 years previously

Sign the FP92A form, available from chemists, for free prescriptions (patients on insulin or an oral hypoglycaemic are eligible). This is sent to the Health Authority, who issues the patient with an exemption certificate

(continued)

Table 6.2. *(continued)*

Administrative tasks *(continued)*

Advise any drivers that they must notify the DVLA in Swansea that they are now a diabetic and record this advice in their notes. Drivers should also be advised to notify their motor insurance company

Recommend joining Diabetes UK, which can advise on various issues, such as insurance

For patients who are started on hypoglycaemic medication, ensure that they always carry instant sugar and a card to indicate that they are diabetic, what treatment they are on and instructions for dealing with hypoglycaemia

Update repeat prescription data and medication review data in the patient record

- Advice:
  1 Give simple explanations of what diabetes is and of its significance.
  2 Encourage the patients to modify any potentially adverse features of their current lifestyles, which includes diet, smoking, alcohol, exercise and foot care.
  3 Give initial advice on self-monitoring.
  4 Explain how the practice organises its care of patients with diabetes.
- Prescription may need to include:
  1 Oral hypoglycaemic drugs or insulin (see *Tables 6.1* and *7.3*).
  2 Testing strips for urine and/or blood.
  3 Syringes, needles, needle clip if on insulin.
- Referral, if indicated, needs to be made to the appropriate hospital outpatient department, podiatrist and/or dietician.
- Investigation(s), see *Table 6.2*.
- Observation requires regular and frequent review until there is stabilisation of blood glucose, risk factors and complications; subsequently, a periodic review (see Chapter 8) is required.

Key Points in this Chapter:

- At diagnosis the answers to the following questions determine the immediate subsequent management:
  1 Is the patient severely ill?
  2 Can this patient be managed in primary care?
  3 What treatment is required to correct blood glucose?

CHAPTER SEVEN

Treatment of Blood Glucose in Type 2 Diabetes

Aiming For Optimal Control

The rationale for optimal glycaemic control is set out in Chapter 3. However, to achieve and maintain the targets (*Table 7.1*) of optimal glycaemic control can be difficult because of the progressive deterioration of pancreatic insulin secretion. Success is possible if the patient, guided and supported by professionals, masters the complex task of balancing self-monitoring, diet, physical activity and blood glucose lowering medication, and if professionals recommend and prescribe appropriate and effective treatment.

Table 7.1. Targets for optimal glycaemic control

Target	Who monitors	Action
Avoiding hypoglycaemia	Patient	Recognises warning signs Balances regular meals, correct dose of therapy and physical activity Able to correct promptly
	Professional	Assesses needs and educates
Fasting blood glucose of 4–7mmol/l	Patient	Able to do and interpret tests Adjusts therapy accordingly
	Professional	Assesses needs and educates
Glycated haemoglobin of less than 7.0%*	Patient	Understands significance of test result Adjusts therapy accordingly
	Professional	Repeats regularly Advises on appropriate therapy changes

*Individualised HbA1c targets should be set between 6.5 and 7.5%; the lower value is preferred for patients at significant risk of vascular complications, the higher for those with limited life expectancy or at risk of iatrogenic hypoglycaemia

Self-monitoring

The achievement of normal blood glucose levels relies upon effective self-monitoring by the patients and/or their carers. The patients need to be motivated, and able to test accurately, interpret the results correctly and act upon them appropriately. To ensure this, patient education is necessary and must be revisited regularly (see Chapter 12).

Blood or urine?

In type 2 diabetes patients who do not require insulin, it may be adequate to test urine for the presence of glucose using test strips, such as Diabur-Test 5000. It is noninvasive, inexpensive and may be preferred by patients who dislike blood testing. However, urine glucose testing has two main limitations:

- The quantity of glucose, if any, in a sample of recently formed urine is more indicative of the mean blood glucose levels over the period of time when the urine was formed than of the blood glucose level at a given moment. Urine levels of glucose do not reflect any sudden fluctuation in blood glucose levels and are, thus, inexact.
- In some type 2 patients, the renal threshold for glycosuria is abnormally high or low. Thus, it is possible for no glucose to be present in the urine with a moderately raised blood glucose level, or for glycosuria to be present with a normal blood glucose level.

Despite these 'disadvantages', if diabetic control is adequate with urine testing (i.e., good HbA1c, infrequent hypoglycaemia), then blood testing may not be necessary in patients on diet alone or oral medication.

Blood glucose testing is recommended for diabetic patients treated with insulin (both types 1 and 2), and may be desirable in patients on diet alone or oral medication who require accurate estimations of their blood glucose. Blood glucose testing is more expensive than urine testing. Correct drawing of blood and use of a properly calibrated machine should produce accurate results. Many varieties of finger-pricking lancets, blood glucose machines and test strips are now available, but only the lancets and strips can be prescribed on an FP10 prescription form. Each different make of blood glucose machine has its own suitable test strips. The current issue of the *Monthly Index of Medical Specialities* (MIMS)[1] lists each make of test strip and the machine(s) each is compatible with. There have been extraordinary technical advances in machines, which now can have sensors that allow the blood drop to be measured outside the machine. Although blood glucose machines are not available on prescription, some are not expensive, costing less than £20. Any blood glucose machine in use must be checked regularly for accuracy. If the GP writes a letter to confirm the diagnosis of diabetes, the patient is exempt from paying Value Added Tax at purchase, provided that the meter is for personal use.

Lancets should be disposed of safely, such as in a needle clipper.

What targets?

Once the patient's diabetic control is stable, the urine should be negative for glucose. If it becomes persistently raised (e.g., more than 2% on four consecutive days) or if the patient becomes ill, professional advice should be sought.

The Diabetes Control and Complications Trial (DCCT) showed that mean blood glucose levels correlate with a given HbA1c level (e.g., HbA1c of 7% correlates with a mean glucose level of 9.5mmol, and rises by 2mmol/l for each increase 1% of Hb1Ac; see Appendix 1).[2] The blood glucose targets for good control are 4–7mmol/l pre-meal and less than 10mmol/l post-meal. If, after stabilisation and despite adjustment of treatment, the blood glucose becomes greater than 20mmol/l for more than 4 days, or if the patient becomes ill, then he or she should consult urgently.

How often and when is testing required?

Testing either the urine or the blood once daily (before different meals and at bedtime) usually suffices for many patients with diabetes. If tight control is less important, the tests can be done less often. However, more frequent testing may be required if the control is poor or if the patient is unwell. Results should be documented in a log that can be brought to the diabetic review.

How to interpret tests

If the test result is regarded as a snapshot of either the period of time when the urine was formed or of the moment the blood sample was taken, it shows the effect of treatment on blood glucose levels. Assuming that the blood glucose level has not been affected by nondiabetic factors, such as other illnesses or medication, persistently abnormal levels should prompt a review of the balance between medication, diet and exercise.

If glycosuria or raised blood glucose is found, an increased dose of either the oral hypoglycaemic drug or insulin may be appropriate. Dietary energy intake, if excessive, should be reduced (see next section). If the oral hypoglycaemic drug or insulin is given in divided doses, the dose that covers the tested time of day must be adjusted accordingly. Patients require education and to develop self-confidence in interpreting and acting upon test results (see later in this chapter for guidance on adjusting insulin doses).

NSF
1
7

Diet or Medical Nutritional Therapy

Medical nutritional therapy (MNT) is an essential component of successful diabetic care. Diabetics no longer need separate or special food. Dietary recommendations for diabetics are virtually the same as those promoted for the general population, but good compliance can produce greater benefits in diabetics, in whom the risk of cardiovascular disease is greater. MNT involves balancing complex issues and needs, tailored to the lifestyle, cultural and religious customs, and to the overall diabetic management of each individual patient.

Goals of medical nutritional therapy in individuals with type 2 diabetes mellitus

The first two goals listed are shared with the general population, and the third is specifically for patients with diabetes:

1 *Provision of essential nutrition.* The optimal diet should supply all the essential nutrients, taking into account the special needs of the patient. Do not forget that type 2 diabetics need the same essential nutrients as the general public.
2 *Prevention of vascular complications.* Appropriate MNT aims to reduce central obesity, improve serum lipid profile and lower blood pressure, all of which are more dangerous in a diabetic.[3]
3. *Adaptation to metabolic problems.* Food intake in type 2 patients must be balanced with exercise and hypoglycaemic treatment (drugs or insulin), so as to avoid the twin perils of hypoglycaemia and hyperglycaemia. Most type 2 patients are overweight, and thus need to reduce their energy intake.

Basic dietary recommendations

General principles

Models of dietary advice

Dieticians no longer recommend 10g carbohydrate exchanges. Instead, appropriate dietary advice should follow a practical model that reflects current dietetic thinking. A synthesis of the two following models may provide a useful basis for dietary advice:

1 'The Balance of Good Health' is a nationally agreed model for dietary advice for patients with diabetes.[4] The model divides foods into five groups:
- Fruit and vegetables – recommends that five portions (400g) are eaten daily;
- Bread, other cereals and potatoes – recommends five portions per day and aims for high-fibre kinds;
- Milk and dairy foods – choose lower fat alternatives;
- Meat, fish and alternatives – aim for smaller portions (a maximum of two portions per day) and lower fat alternatives;
- Fatty and sugary foods – aim to reduce quantities.

2 'The Healthy Eating Pyramid' is a visual way to help translate dietary advice into practical eating habits.[5] Foods are divided into three strata based upon what proportion of a healthy diabetic diet they should constitute:
- Consume sparingly: eat minimum amounts of fats, alcohol and sugars (e.g., cakes, fried food, savoury snacks, processed meat, honey, diabetes 'specialist' foods);
- Consume in moderation: eat small servings of protein foods (e.g., lean meat, fish, eggs, low-fat dairy products);
- Consume as the basis of diet: eat mainly foods rich in starch (e.g. vegetables, beans, fresh fruit, wholemeal bread, pasta, rice).

Delivering dietary advice

In undertaking dietary counselling, the professional assumes responsibility for the process and is well advised to proceed through the following stages:
- Assessment of the patient's current diet, and readiness for and barriers to change (a model of change is discussed in Chapter 12);
- Discussion and negotiation of possible changes;
- Setting goals that are patient-centred and realistic;
- Monitoring the patient's progress at suitably regular intervals and maintaining support.

While adhering to the same models and counselling process that suit the general population, with particular emphasis on reducing cardiovascular risk, diabetic dietetic advice should emphasise the need to space regular meals and snacks appropriately throughout the day. This will spread nutrient intake and avoid hypoglycaemia. Patients should be warned to avoid special diabetic products, which are expensive and usually high in fat.

Specific food types

Dietary energy and body weight

If the BMI is greater than 25 and the patient has intra-abdominal fat accumulation, then dietary advice should aim for reduced energy intake and for weight loss.[3,6] Patients should be advised to reduce their consumption of energy-dense foods, particularly fat and alcohol. Detailed guidance on energy intake is not needed if the BMI is within an acceptable range, between 19 and 25.

Protein

Protein is an essential nutrient that provides amino acids for new tissue formation. Protein intake should constitute 15–20% of total energy intake (optimally 0.8g/kg body weight/day). Excessive intake of protein (more than 20% of total energy intake) is neither necessary nor advisable. Cereal foods, soya products, tofu, quorn and pulses add considerably to the protein content of the diet.

Moderate hyperglycaemia can cause increased protein turnover, but, since most adults eat at least 50% more protein than required, intake should not be increased. Modification of protein intake is unnecessary if renal function is within the normal range. If there is renal impairment, then protein restriction and other dietary modifications should only be undertaken under the supervision of a suitably qualified dietician.

Fat

The following are important points that should be borne in mind (see also Chapter 8, in particular the discussion on lipids):

- Saturated fat is the main dietary determinant of serum low-density lipoprotein (LDL) cholesterol levels.
- In most European countries, current intake of saturated fat is above the recommended maximum 10% of total energy intake.
- Diabetics appear to be more sensitive to dietary cholesterol than the rest of the population. Three food groups are particularly high in cholesterol: eggs, offal and shellfish.
- *Trans*-unsaturated fatty acids (often found in manufactured confectionery products and some margarine) and *N*-6-polyunsaturated fatty acids raise plasma LDL cholesterol. The former also lower plasma high-density lipoprotein (HDL) cholesterol.
- Diets low in saturated fat and high in carbohydrate or enriched in mono-unsaturated fatty acids with a *cis*-configuration (see *Table 7.2* for examples) lower serum LDL cholesterol levels.
- *N*-3-polyunsaturated fatty acids are found in foods such as oil-rich fish (mackerel, herring, sardines, pilchards, trout and mullet). *N*-3-polyunsaturated fatty acid supplements have been shown to lower plasma triglyceride levels in type 2 diabetics, but they raise serum LDL cholesterol levels.
- Reduced fat diets, when maintained over the long term, can help to bring about a modest weight loss and an improvement in dyslipidaemia.
- Regular use of foods with fat replacers and/or substitutes is safe and may help to reduce saturated fat and cholesterol intake, but will not reduce total energy intake or weight.

Table 7.2. Examples of foods with particular characteristics[3]

Food type	Examples
Contains mono-unsaturated fatty acids	Cashew nuts, hazelnuts, almonds, herring, salmon, pilchards, mullet, peanut butter, olive oil, rapeseed oil, goose fat, avocado
Carbohydrates with a low glycaemic index and/or rich in soluble fibre	Buckwheat, rice, oats, pasta, kidney beans, soybeans, chickpeas, apples, oranges, milk
Rich in antioxidants	Carrots, corn oil, potatoes, tomatoes, broccoli, peas, spinach, oranges, milk, pineapples

Recommendations to achieve the main goals (to limit saturated fat and dietary cholesterol intake) are:

- Less than 10% of energy intake should be from saturated fats. If the serum LDL cholesterol is greater than 2.60mmol/l proportion, this should be reduced to less than 7% if weight loss is desirable or replaced with either carbohydrate or mono-unsaturated fat if weight is to be maintained.
- Dietary cholesterol intake should be less than 300mg/day. If the serum LDL cholesterol is greater than 2.60mmol/l, this should be reduced to less than 200mg/day.
- The intake of *trans*-unsaturated fatty acids and *N*-6-polyunsaturated fatty acids should be minimised.

Carbohydrate

The basic concepts for carbohydrates are:

- When referring to carbohydrate, the terms *sugars, starch* and *fibre* are preferred to the terms *simple sugars, complex* and *fast-acting carbohydrates,* as the latter are not well defined.
- Carbohydrate exchange systems based upon 10g portions do not improve glycaemic control and are no longer used.
- Many factors (including type of sugar, nature of starch, method of food processing and cooking, food form, other food components, blood glucose levels, severity of glucose intolerance) can affect patients' glycaemic response to foods.
- The total amount of carbohydrate in the dietary intake seems to be more important than the source or type.
- Intake of foods with a low 'glycaemic index' (GI) has not been shown to improve glycaemic control in type 2 diabetics, but may improve the lipid profile.
- Consumption of the sugar sucrose does not increase glycaemia more than isocaloric amounts of starch.
- Fibre-containing foods, such as whole grains, fruit and vegetables, provide vitamins, minerals and other substances important for good health. However, both diabetic and nondiabetic individuals would need to consume very large amounts of fibre (how palatable?) to produce metabolic improvements on glycaemia and lipid profiles.
- Intake of foods that contain naturally occurring resistant starch (corn starch) may modify post-prandial glycaemic response and reduce more extreme fluctuations in blood glucose levels, but there is no published evidence of long-term benefits to diabetics.

Recommendations for carbohydrates are:

- When calculating optimal intake, greater attention should be paid to the total amount of carbohydrate than to its source or type.
- Foods with carbohydrate from fibre-rich foods (whole grains, fruit and vegetables) and from low-fat milk should be included in the diet. There is no evidence to support increasing fibre intake in diabetics above the levels recommended for the rest of the population.
- Sucrose or sucrose-containing foods should not be restricted for diabetics, but can be used in substitution for other carbohydrate sources in the context of a healthy diet with appropriate hypoglycaemic medication cover.
- The expert consensus is that carbohydrate and mono-unsaturated fat together should provide 60–70% of energy intake, but precise and relative proportions may vary according to individual factors, such as age, activity levels and weight.

Alcoholic drinks

The same precautions regarding alcoholic drinks in the general population apply to patients with type 2 diabetes, that is to stay within the recommended limits, avoid drinking on an empty stomach or as a substitute for a meal, and to remember that low-carbohydrate beers are higher in alcohol and calories. In patients with type 2 diabetes, drinking two to three glasses of wine (or the equivalent quantity of beer) may produce an insignificant drop in blood glucose, but does not increase the risk of hypoglycaemia.[7] Alcohol is potentially a major energy source, but it can contribute to elevated blood pressure and serum triglycerides. To reduce the risk of significant hypoglycaemia in type 2 patients treated with sulphonylureas or insulin, alcohol should be consumed with foods that contain carbohydrate.

Micronutrients

Diabetics should be educated both about the importance of consuming adequate quantities of vitamins and minerals from natural sources and about the potential toxicity of very large doses of these in supplements. Supplementation is indicated only in selected patient groups (e.g., elderly, those on restricted calorie diets and those with proved deficiency).

Since diabetics may be in a 'state of increased oxidative stress', there has been considerable interest in exploring the benefits of antioxidant vitamin supplementation. However, as yet there is no placebo-controlled trial evidence of benefit, but adverse effects may occur.

Other circumstances

Older adults

There is limited evidence on the changing nutritional needs of older diabetics, but they have lower energy requirements than younger adults. Undernutrition is more likely than overnutrition, and therefore caution is required when prescribing a weight-loss diet. When evaluating involuntary weight loss in the elderly, the clinician should consider the possibility of undernutrition. Suitable physical activity should be encouraged.

Hypertension

The MNT management of hypertension should focus upon weight reduction and restriction of sodium intake, both of which lower blood pressure. The ADA's Expert Consensus recommends that the maximum daily intake of sodium should be 2400mg (100mmol), or of salt (sodium chloride) it should be 6000mg.[6]

Also, chronic excessive alcohol consumption (greater than 30–60g per day or greater than 4 units per day) is associated with raised blood pressure, and should be reduced.

Vegetarians

- Lacto-ovo vegetarians eat no meat or fish, but take eggs, milk and milk products;
- Lacto vegetarians take only milk and milk products;
- Vegans eat no animal foods.

Different ethnic groups

The aims and basic recommendations outlined above are appropriate for all diabetics, irrespective of the cultural customs, religious affiliation or ethnic origin of the patient. The professional needs to tailor the advice given within the bounds of what is acceptable, attractive and realistic. Different Indo-Asian diets are suitable, provided that *total fat intake is reduced*.

The manner in which food is prepared is important. While patients are encouraged to substitute olive oil for ghee in cooking, quantities should be measured and minimised. It is also desirable to reduce the consumption of gur, jaggery, honey (too much sugar), samosas, bhajis, puris (too much fat), jelabi, laddo, burfi, gulab jamen and kulfi. For curries, it is recommended to fry off spices and drain excess fat, and then make the curry in the normal way.

Referral to dietician

Practice nurses and GPs are ideally placed to provide the basics of sound nutritional advice and should reinforce this as appropriate when reviews are undertaken. However, a referral to a qualified dietician for an individual dietary assessment is appropriate:

- When type 2 diabetes is diagnosed;
- When insulin is started;
- When other medical problems are present (e.g., obesity, hyperlipidaemia, renal impairment);
- When glycated haemoglobin remains persistently raised;
- If the patient fails to achieve or maintain optimal body weight.

Oral Drug Therapy: An Overview

From diagnosis, both patient and professional need to be aware that there is likely to be a progressive deterioration over time of pancreatic beta cell function, as a result of which most type 2 diabetics eventually require insulin to achieve acceptable glycaemic control. The choice of treatment should follow a 'step-up' policy, summarised in *Table 7.3*. The main classes of medications that lower oral blood glucose act by improving either insulin secretion or insulin action. For a drug to stimulate insulin secretion, it is necessary that the pancreatic beta cells be functioning still. Further details about the drug classes discussed below can be found in the *British National Formulary* (BNF; Chapter 6, section 1.2).[8]

The combination of self-monitoring results, a recent glycated haemoglobin result and the patient's well-being should guide both dose changes and decisions about additional medication (or step-up). The interval between any dose changes must allow sufficient time for their effect to be established, but prompt action is indicated in the event of repeated hypoglycaemia or significant hyperglycaemia. Ideally, additional medication should be introduced only after the maximum recommended dose of current medication has failed to achieve reasonable glycaemic control or is not tolerated.

New drugs, some with different modes of action, have been introduced recently or are due for imminent launch in the UK and European markets. With the availability of longer-term surveillance and efficacy data and with increased clinician experience, the role of these new drugs will be defined more precisely in the future.

Whatever drug therapy is prescribed, it should be combined with interventions aimed at optimising lifestyle (see the previous section, Diet or medical nutrition therapy, and Chapter 8). A patient's compliance with treatment needs to be discussed and monitored if glycaemic control appears problematic. Other medical problems must be managed appropriately. If uncertain about any aspect of management, it is sensible to seek specialist help.

Table 7.3. Summary of the treatment of raised blood glucose in type 2 diabetes

Step	Evaluation	Intervention
1	Ketonuria absent Fasting blood glucose is <15mmol/l	Dietary advice
2a	Ketonuria absent Fasting blood glucose is >15mmol/l or failure of diet to control blood glucose Obese (BMI >25kg/cm^2) Absence of renal (creatinine >130nmol/l), hepatic or cardiac impairment *or* risk of sudden deterioration	Metformin
2b	As in step 2a, but nonobese or intolerant of metformin	Insulin secretagogue [sulphonylurea *or* meglitinide* (especially if fasting)]
3a	Ketonuria absent Failure of first-line drug to control blood glucose Absence of renal, hepatic or cardiac impairment	Combination of metformin *and* insulin secretagogue
3b	Ketonuria absent Failure of metformin and sulphonylurea combination to control blood glucose Absence of renal, hepatic or cardiac impairment Intolerance of either first-line drug	Combination of thiazolidinedione *and* metformin (preferable) or sulphonylurea
4	Failure to control blood glucose with oral agents	Insulin, *with or without* metformin (in the absence of renal, hepatic or cardiac impairment) *or* sulphonylurea

*Repaglinide can be prescribed either as monotherapy or in combination with metformin, but currently nateglinide is licensed only in combination with metformin.

Insulin Secretagogues

There are two main groups: the longer-established *sulphonylureas* and the recently introduced rapid-acting insulin secretagogues repaglinide and nateglinide. NICE's *Clinical Guidelines* recommend that 'a generic sulphonylurea should normally be the insulin secretagogue of choice'.[9]

Sulphonylureas

The sulphonylurea drugs act by stimulating insulin secretion from beta cells (although there is less stimulation of first-phase secretion than by the meglitinide class discussed below), but do not affect insulin resistance. Sulphonylureas can encourage weight gain in the obese and can cause hypoglycaemia. In the absence of ketonuria, sulphonylureas are indicated in nonobese patients whose blood glucose is not controlled by diet. There are several to choose from, all of which have comparable blood glucose lowering effects, but with different durations of action. Short-acting sulphonylureas are safer and, thus, preferred in the elderly. All sulphonylureas should be introduced slowly and the dose titrated according to the results of urine or blood tests.

Tolbutamide

Tolbutamide is short acting and inexpensive. It is available in 500mg tablets. The starting dose is one-half tablet before breakfast, up to a maximum of 2g per day in divided doses.

Gliclazide

Gliclazide (Diamicron) is excreted in bile, and thus is suitable for patients with renal impairment. It is more expensive than tolbutamide and is available in 80mg tablets. The starting dose is one-half tablet once daily, up to a maximum of two tablets twice daily (320mg). Up to 160mg can be given as a single dose. A 'modified release' formulation of gliclazide, called Diamicron MR, became available recently. It has the same duration of action, but its improved bioavailability allows once-daily dosing and the dose has been reduced from 80mg to 30mg per tablet. It is more expensive.

Glipizide

Glipizide (Glibenese, Minodiab) has a range of action similar to that of gliclazide, but it is cleared by the kidneys. The tablets are available in 2.5mg and 5mg tablets. The starting dose is 2.5–5mg once daily, up to 15mg per day as a single dose and a maximum of 40mg per day in divided doses. A longer-acting formulation of glipizide may soon be available.

Glimepiride

Glimepiride (Amaryl) is a new-generation sulphonylurea; its manufacturers claim that it stimulates a more physiological insulin release with a lower risk of hypoglycaemia. It is taken once daily and is available in 1mg, 2mg, 3mg and 4mg tablets. 1mg of glimepiride is the equivalent of 80mg of gliclazide. The dose range is from 1 to 6 mg daily. It can be combined with basal (intermediate- or long-acting) insulin, unlike other sulphonylureas.

Others

Both glibenclamide and chlorpropamide are longer acting and can induce hypoglycaemic episodes, especially in the elderly. Chlorpropamide interacts with alcohol. The author would not recommend either drug, particularly as superior alternative sulphonylureas are now available.

New formulations that modify the duration of action of the sulphonylureas gliclazide, glipizide and glibenclamide have been or are in the process of being launched.

Meglitinide analogues

Meglitinide analogues [post-prandial glucose regulators (PPRGs) or rapid-acting insulin secretagogues] also stimulate insulin release by the pancreas. PPRGs are best initiated at an earlier stage in the disease process, when pancreatic beta cells still have a reasonable capacity to secrete insulin. The main action of PPRGs is to increase early (first-phase) insulin secretion in response to rising plasma glucose levels by pancreatic beta cells, and so reduce the mealtime 'glucose spike'. In contrast, sulphonylureas have less effect on this first phase. PPRGs have a quicker onset and shorter duration of action than sulphonylureas. PPRGs may prove preferable to sulphonylureas in a type 2 diabetic who either needs to fast (e.g., Muslims during Ramadan) or whose meal times are unpredictable and/or irregular.

Repaglinide

Repaglinide (NovoNorm) was launched in 1998 in the UK. It has a rapid onset of action (peak level at 50 minutes after administration) and is short-acting (duration of 3 hours). The initial dose is 0.5mg, usually taken within 15 minutes before each main meal. The dose can be increased at intervals of 1–2 weeks to a maximum of 4mg per single dose and 16mg per day. It is licensed for use either as monotherapy or in combination with metformin. It is contraindicated in severe hepatic or renal impairment, and reported side effects include visual disturbances, gastrointestinal symptoms and rash. Both hypoglycaemia and weight gain are possible risks with repaglinide, although the risks are less than with sulphonylureas.

Nateglinide

Nateglinide (Starlix) is an amino acid derivative, launched in the UK in 2001. When administered pre-prandially, it produces an 'insulinotropic' response (dependent upon the amount of glucose that enters the blood) within 15 minutes. Nateglinide appears to have a slighter quicker onset and shorter duration of action than repaglinide. The initial dose is 60mg, rising to 180mg, three times daily, taken 1 to 30 minutes before a meal. Nateglinide is contraindicated in severe liver disease and pregnancy. Currently, it is licensed for prescription only in combination with metformin. Nateglinide interacts with ACE inhibitors, diuretics and corticosteroids. It produces minimal weight gain and has a lower risk of causing hypoglycaemia, but this is still possible in elderly patients and in those with adrenal or pituitary insufficiency.

Drugs that Improve Insulin Action

Biguanides

Metformin (Glucophage) is the only available drug in this class. It is the first-choice drug for obese type 2 patients, but it is an option for first-line therapy in the nonobese, and it can be combined with all secretagogues, both glitazones and the different insulins. It is available in 500 and 850mg tablets. The starting dose can be 250–500mg after main meals, followed by stepped increases to a maximum of 2g per day in divided doses. Metformin works by decreasing gluconeogenesis in the liver and by increasing glucose uptake in peripheral tissues. Its excretion is entirely renal and it has a short half life. Its main side effects are on the gastrointestinal tract, and they can be lessened by a stepped approach to increasing the dose and by the dose being taken with or after food. Metformin does not result in either weight gain or serious hypoglycaemia. Strict adherence to all the published contraindications, related to a perceived increased risk of precipitating lactic acidosis (not supported by systemic reviews[10]), would result in metformin being prescribed only rarely, despite its undoubted value to many type 2 diabetics in achieving glycaemic control and reducing vascular risk. Revised specific contraindications and guidelines for withdrawing metformin have been suggested recently:[11]

- Stop if the serum creatinine is greater than 150µmols/l (less if elderly);

- Withdraw during periods of suspected tissue hypoxia (e.g., through myocardial infarction or sepsis);
- Withdraw for 3 days after contrast medium that contains iodine has been given and reinstate when renal function is normal and stable;
- Withdraw 2 days before general anaesthesia and reinstate when renal function is normal and stable.

Thiazolidinediones

Thiazolidinediones (TZDs), also known as glitazones or peroxisome proliferator-activated receptor-gamma (PPAR-γ) agonists,[12] act by promoting glucose utilisation peripherally, which enhances insulin action, but does not affect insulin secretion. They are thought both to activate receptors, located mainly in adipose tissue, that affect glucose and lipid metabolism and to maintain insulin secretion by pancreatic beta cells,[13] because they reduce the effect of glucose 'toxicity'.

In October 1997, troglitazone was launched in the UK and was voluntarily withdrawn by its manufacturers weeks later, following reports of serious hepatic reactions worldwide.

Rosiglitazone and pioglitazone

Rosiglitazone (Avandia) and pioglitazone (Actos) are two newer and more potent agents, which have been available in the USA since 1999, and were launched in the UK during 2000. Current evidence suggests that neither agent causes hepatic impairment. In the USA both drugs are licensed for monotherapy or in combination with either metformin or sulphonylureas, and pioglitazone can be used in combination with insulin. However, in Europe they are licensed for treatment *only in combination* with either metformin or sulphonylureas, but not as part of triple therapy or in combination with insulin. Rosiglitazone is available as 4mg and 8mg tablets. Its initial dose is 4mg once daily, increasing to 8mg daily, either in single or two divided doses after 8 weeks, depending upon response. Pioglitazone is available as 15mg and 30mg tablets. The initial dose is 15mg once daily, but can be increased to 30mg once daily. After starting either drug, there may be a delay of 6–10 weeks before their full effect is seen. Both glitazones are very expensive when compared to metformin or to most sulphonylureas.

The NICE Appraisal Committee issued guidance in 2000/1 (the review is due to be published in 2003) on the use of both rosiglitazone and pioglitazone within their current UK licences:[14,15]

- Glitazone combination therapy with a first-line drug (as an alternative to insulin) should be offered to patients unable to take or tolerate metformin and sulphonylurea as a combination therapy, or in whom this combination does not achieve adequate glycaemic control after an adequate trial.
- It is preferable to combine a glitazone with metformin than with a sulphonylurea, particularly if the patient is obese.
- Liver function [looking for a threefold rise in alanine transferase (ALT)] should be checked before starting a glitazone, approximately bimonthly in the first year of use, and 'periodically' afterwards.

Adherence to the NICE guidelines is usually recommended, but readers should bear in mind two situations in which this guidance may not always be the optimal way to improve glycaemic control:

- In obese type 2 patients (particularly from some ethnic groups), insulin resistance is likely to be significant. Tackling this by a combination of nonpharmacological (improving diet and levels of physical activity) and pharmacological interventions is, therefore, a priority. If monotherapy with metformin fails to achieve adequate glycaemic control (step 2a in *Table 7.3*), then, as the next step (3b), combination with a glitazone may be preferred to an insulin secretagogue. The rationale here is that a sulphonylurea potentially causes weight gain and so may be less helpful than a glitazone that acts to reduce insulin resistance.
- The NICE guidelines warn that the substitution of a glitazone for a first-line drug, after failure of the metformin–sulphonylurea combination, does risk an initial worsening of glycaemic control. However, this may not always be recoverable. Introducing insulin at this stage may be preferable to the substitution of a glitazone.

Further evidence from long-term data is needed to define more precisely the role glitazones can play in diabetes care, not only in overall glycaemic control (by delaying the introduction of insulin), but also in the reduction of vascular risk; as yet, no studies have been published to show whether these drugs reduce vascular complications. Short-term data suggest that both drugs may have some blood pressure lowering effect, and that neither has an adverse

Table 7.4. Overview of insulin preparations[5]

Category	Generic types	Examples	Onset of action (minutes)	Peak of action	Duration of action (hours)
Rapid acting		Lispro, aspart	10–20	40–60 minutes	3–5
Short acting	Regular*	Actrapid, Humulin S	15–60	1–3 hours	4–8
Short–intermediate acting (biphasic)	Regular – isophane (NPH) mixture	Mixtard, Humulin M1 to M5	15–60	2 peaks (as for its components)	12–18
Intermediate acting (Basal)	Isophane (NPH)	Insulatard, Humulin I	60–120	4–8 hours	12–18
Long acting	Crystalline zinc suspensions	Ultratard, Humulin Zn	120–240	6–18 hours	18–24+
Prolonged acting		Insulin glargine	90	Plateau	24

*The term 'soluble' no longer applies to short-acting insulins only, since prolonged preparations (such as insulin glargine) have become available.

effect on lipid profiles. Indeed, the NICE guidance cites evidence that HDL cholesterol levels increase and triglyceride levels fall when 30mg or more of pioglitazone are used. Both drugs can cause weight gain, in part through fluid retention, which may precipitate heart failure, particularly if a glitazone is combined with insulin. The current licence of these drugs may alter in the future, as further data become available on their safety and on the potential benefit of their use as monotherapy (with the theoretical advantage of earlier use), in combination with other agents, such as repaglinide and insulin, or as part of triple therapy.

Other Oral Drug Therapy

Alpha-glucosidase inhibitors

The only drug in this class currently available in the UK is acarbose (Glucobay). It inhibits intestinal alpha-glucosidase, and so delays the digestion of starch and sucrose, which increase blood glucose levels after ingestion of carbohydrate. The result is a fall in post-prandial glucose and insulin levels. Acarbose can be prescribed either as monotherapy or in combination with other oral agents. It does not cause weight gain and is unlikely to cause hypoglycaemia as monotherapy. Unfortunately, its widespread use is limited by its gastrointestinal side effects (which occur in up to 60% of patients). These are dose dependent, and include flatulence, bloating and diarrhoea. As these occur most frequently at the initiation of treatment, careful titration may reduce their incidence. Acarbose is best taken with meals rich in starch. Acarbose is available in 50mg and 100mg tablets. The starting dose is 50mg once daily just prior to or during the first mouthful of food. The dose can be increased to 50mg three times daily, and eventually up to a maximum of 200mg three times daily. It should be considered as an alternative in patients unable to use the other oral drugs. Acarbose is expensive.

Insulin

Clinical indications for changing to insulin in type 2 diabetes

Since pancreatic beta secretion declines as the duration of their illness increases, most type 2 diabetics eventually need to be transferred onto insulin. Clear, calm and prior explanation should prevent patients who arrive at this point from feeling that they have 'failed' or are to blame.

This transfer should be considered in any of the following circumstances:

- Intolerance of and/or inadequate response to oral hypoglycaemic agents;
- Contraindications to oral therapy (e.g., metformin and renal impairment, rosiglitazone and hepatic impairment);
- Acute symptoms of hyperglycaemia or intercurrent illness and/or steroid therapy, which can exacerbate hyperglycaemia;
- Continual weight loss (in the presence or absence of ketones);
- Poor healing and/or recurrent infections;
- Postmyocardial infarction;
- Pregnancy.

Insulin preparations

The variety of insulin preparations currently available is bewildering. Insulins can be classified according to their onset and duration of action, summarised in *Table 7.4*. They also vary according to their origin and method of manufacture (animal-derived, semisynthetic or synthetic), modifications that alter the duration of action, and their mode of delivery (e.g., syringe, pen, infusion device – see below).

Onset and duration of action

Different pharmaceutical companies have adopted different names for the same insulins or their mixtures. Further details are available in the latest BNF (Section 6.1.1) or MIMS:[1,8]

- *Rapid-acting insulins.* Two preparations are available currently, lispro and aspart. Their onset is quick (within 5–10 minutes), their peak of action is early (within 1 hour) and their duration of action is brief (3–5 hours). The optimal time to inject is just as a meal begins. These insulins are particularly used in a basal bolus regimen (see below).
- *Short-acting insulins.* Many preparations are available. Ideally, short-acting insulin should be given 30–45 minutes before meals to match its peak action to glucose absorption from the gastrointestinal tract. A delayed meal risks hypoglycaemia and injecting just before, during or after a meal does not facilitate tight glycaemic control. In these circumstances, rapid-acting insulin may be more suitable.
- *Intermediate-acting insulins.* The widely used isophane preparations (also known as neutral protamine Hagedorn, NPH) are complexes of insulin and protamine. Although these can be used as monotherapy either once or twice daily, they are often mixed with either rapid- or short-acting insulins, or, when given as a single bedtime dose, combined with daytime oral agents (see below). For convenience, premixed insulins (also known as biphasic) are available, and contain both short- or rapid-acting and intermediate-acting insulins (e.g., Mixtard, Humulin M, and Humalog Mix) in various proportions. European nomenclature states the short-acting percentage before the intermediate-acting percentage. The 30/70 mixture is often favoured in the UK.
- *Long-acting insulins.* These are becoming less popular, because their mixture with short-acting insulins causes problems, and because premixed and prolonged-acting analogue insulins have now become available and are being used increasingly.

Origin and method of manufacture

Short-, intermediate- and long-acting insulins are either based on the human sequence of amino acids or extracted from an animal pancreas, usually porcine (less antigenic than beef), and then purified. Synthetic human insulin is produced either by enzyme modification of porcine insulin (emp) or, more commonly, from a proinsulin synthesised by bacteria (prb) or from a precursor synthesised by yeast (pyr), using recombinant DNA technology. Human insulins have a more rapid onset and shorter duration of activity than porcine insulins.[16]

Modifications that alter the onset and duration of action

Recently, genetically engineered insulin analogues that contain modifications to soluble human insulin have been introduced. These include:

- Rapid-acting, such as lispro (transposes two amino acids, lysine and praline, on the B chain to B28 lysine and B29 proline) and aspart (aspartate replaces praline at B28).

- Prolonged-acting, such as insulin glargine (two additional arginine molecules are placed at B31 and B32, at the C terminus of the B chain, and arginine replaces asparagines at A21 – the latter makes the molecule more stable). Insulin glargine was launched in the UK in 2002. Its onset is at about 90 minutes and its duration is 24 hours or longer, with a prolonged plateau of concentration rather than a peak. Its manufacturers claim that this absence of a peak reduces the risk of nocturnal hypoglycaemia. Thus, insulin glargine should be used as once-daily basal insulin administered in the evening or at bedtime, either on its own or in combination with metformin, glimepiride or short- or rapid-acting insulin (see below). A NICE technology appraisal published at the end of 2002 does not recommend the routine use of insulin glargine in people with type 2 diabetes, except in the following groups:[17]
  - those who require assistance by a carer or health care professional to administer their insulin injections;
  - those whose lifestyle is restricted significantly by recurrent symptomatic hypoglycaemic episodes;
  - those who would otherwise need twice-daily basal insulin injections in combination with oral hypoglycaemic agents (see Regimen 4 below).

When converting to insulin glargine, the dosage should be 20% less than the total 24 hour dose of the previous basal insulin.

Possible insulin regimens

The insulin regimen used has to be tailored to the patient's needs and lifestyle, and it must take into account the patient's wishes and sensitivities. Rapid-, short-, intermediate- and long-acting insulin preparations may be injected either separately or mixed together in the same syringe. A variety of regimens are available, some of which are discussed here.

Regimen one

The most popular regimen is to stop all oral hypoglycaemic agents (except metformin) and give *twice daily insulin before meals in the morning and evening*. The basis of this regimen is intermediate-acting insulin (often two-thirds of the total daily dose is given before breakfast and one-third before the evening meal or at bedtime); however, this is often given in combination with a short-acting insulin, either drawn up separately or as a pre-mixed combination. In some circumstances, better glycaemic control is achieved using different preparations for the morning and evening injections. The conventional practice is to begin at a dose of 8–10 units twice daily, with gradual increases in dose until the glycaemic targets are reached. However, the titration of insulin doses to reach normoglycaemia can be accelerated by using slide rules, devised by the UKPDS and now available to health care professionals. These slide rules calculate the total insulin dose likely to be required by any diabetic, based upon gender, fasting blood glucose, height and weight. The doses are recommended for both short-acting (prandial) and intermediate-acting (basal) insulins, usually given twice daily as a mixture. The initial day's total insulin dose should be one-half to two-thirds of the calculated likely final total insulin dose. The drawback of the slide rule and an accelerated increase of insulin dose is greater weight gain as compared to the conventional slower insulin dose titration.

Regimen two

Once-daily insulin (a basal insulin, such as an intermediate-acting isophane) may be appropriate for those patients (e.g., a frail, isolated elderly diabetic) for whom tight blood glucose control is not the main therapeutic goal or hypoglycaemia may be disastrous. Insulin glargine may prove a more useful alternative in this group. Not only is it possible to combine met-formin with the first three of the insulin regimens described to overcome insulin resistance, but also there is good evidence that better glycaemic control, weight loss and reduced risk of hypoglycaemia are more likely when using a metformin and insulin combination.

Regimen three

Basal bolus regimen, with a *rapid-acting insulin three times daily* before breakfast, midday and the evening meal, with either *twice-daily intermediate-acting* or *a single injection of pro-longed-acting insulin* (e.g., insulin glargine) *at bedtime*. If using Humalog Mix (rapid- and intermediate-acting insulin mixture) twice daily, it may still be appropriate to give an addi-tional dose of rapid-acting insulin (i.e., lispro) to cover a large meal.

Regimen four

Combination of an intermediate-acting or prolonged-acting insulin once daily at bedtime and oral hypoglycaemic drug(s) during the day (a sulphonylurea, such as glimepiride), when the oral combination of a hypoglycaemic drug (other than metformin) with a sulphonylurea has failed to achieve satisfactory glycaemic control (step 3b in *Table 7.3*). This regimen has not been shown to be more effective than insulin alone, but the combination may be more prac-tical for some patients. The suitable starting dose of basal insulin can be calculated using the slide rule referred to above.

Insulin dose adjustment

Insulin doses need to be titrated against blood glucose levels, aiming for 4–7mmol/l before meals, as set out in *Table 7.1*. It may take a few weeks to achieve normal blood glucose levels.

Principles of dose adjustment

No single set of advice copes with every situation. However, a number of guiding principles may help:

- Avoid changing insulin on the basis of a one-off reading;
- Review monitoring and injection techniques, eating and activity levels and patterns;
- Consider the category, dose and injection timing of the insulin used;
- Look for patterns, such as periods of day with the greatest problems;
- Agree finite dose changes, such as two units, and allow an interval of a few days between dose changes to give time for the patient to adapt.

Twice-daily regimen (free-mixing regime)

- If glucose is high or low *before breakfast*, increase or decrease *evening long-acting* insulin;
- If glucose is high or low *before lunch*, increase or decrease *morning short-acting* insulin;
- If glucose is high or low *before supper*, increase or decrease *morning long-acting* insulin;
- If glucose is high or low *before bed*, increase or decrease *evening short-acting* insulin.

Twice-daily regimen (fixed biphasic insulin regime)

- If glucose is high or low *before breakfast*, increase or decrease *evening* insulin dose;
- If glucose is high or low *before supper*, increase or decrease *morning* insulin dose;
- Other adjustments probably require a change in the mixture's components.

Basal bolus regimen
- If glucose is high or low *before breakfast*, increase or decrease *evening long-acting* insulin;
- If glucose is high or low *before lunch*, increase or decrease *morning rapid-acting* insulin;
- If glucose is high or low *before supper*, increase or decrease *lunchtime rapid-acting* insulin;
- If glucose is high or low *before bed*, increase or decrease *teatime rapid-acting* insulin.

Over insulinisation
Recurrent hypoglycaemia, weight gain, wildly variable blood glucose values and subtle features of chronic hypoglycaemia (headache, personality change in elderly, the need to eat) suggest a chronic overdose of insulin.

How to make the change to insulin
It may be best to seek the advice of the hospital diabetic clinic or a diabetes specialist nurse before initiating insulin. Unless the patient is ill, insulin can be started on an outpatient basis. The initiation of insulin requires that the professional responsible has the appropriate knowledge and skills, that sufficient time is available to address all of the patient's needs and agenda (ideas, concerns and expectations) and that the professional remains accessible to monitor progress and provide support.

If the primary care team takes charge, an agreed and effective protocol should be followed. Success is possible: in the author's practice, the average glycated haemoglobin (HbA1c) of the first 15 patients transferred onto insulin dropped from 9.7 to 6.9%.[18] Some innovatory teams have looked at a group approach, in which 6–10 patients can attend together, with the benefits of increased cost-effectiveness and of greater mutual support between often-anxious individuals in a similar situation.

In assessing the person who requires insulin, the following issues should be considered:
- *Implications to lifestyle.* Patients who switch to insulin are no longer eligible for a group 2 driving licence (bus, coach and large goods vehicle driver). Switching to insulin may affect the employment circumstances of those in the police, fire services and armed forces.
- *Level of support at home.* This is particularly important if dexterity and/or vision are impaired and the patient may not be able to administer his or her own insulin.
- *Cultural and religious beliefs.* For example, animal-derived insulins are unacceptable to Muslims, Jews and strict vegans. The insulin regimen used must avoid hypoglycaemia when the patient is required to fast. Clear and effective communication must be based on the languages used by the patient and/or carer. Any written material used must be appropriate for the level of literacy of the patient and/or carer.
- *Psychological and physical health issues.* In very obese insulin-resistant patients, insulin may cause further weight gain. Many type 2 diabetics who switch to insulin may be frightened of needles and may regard the switch as a 'failure'. A clear explanation of the likely benefits that arise from good diabetic control with a demonstration using a syringe or pen may go some way to alleviating these fears. Continuity of care helps: the health care professional involved should be prepared to offer future advice and support.

Key educational points
Clear and correct advice on the following aspects of self-administering insulin should be given to patients, along and suitable written literature should be made available for reference.[19]

Equipment: choosing a suitable injection device

The choice is between a disposable U100 insulin syringe with an attached needle and one of the bewilderingly wide ranges of pen-injector devices. Both have their respective advantages and disadvantages. Staying in touch with a friendly diabetes specialist nurse should enable the primary care team to keep up-to-date with developments. MIMS[1] is a useful source of information about the syringes, pen needles and most pens that are available free on FP10 prescription. Syringes are smaller and lighter than pens, but pens are more portable, may be more suitable for those with visual problems and the patient does not need to carry a vial of insulin to be drawn up for each injection. Both syringes and pens require some degree of manual dexterity to use.

Mixing insulins

If free mixing insulins, the short-acting preparation must be drawn into the syringe *before* the intermediate-acting preparation to avoid contamination of the short-acting vial with protamine or zinc.

Injection technique

The injection technique is as important as the type of insulin injected or the device used. The three key factors that influence insulin absorption are depth, site and technique (*Table 7.5*):

- Subcutaneous depth is preferred for everyday use, but the distribution of subcutaneous tissue can vary between ages, sex, body mass distribution and site. Appropriate needle size is important to avoid the injection being either too shallow (intradermal) or too deep (intramuscular or another structure).
- Sites should be rotated and, for reliable absorption, different areas should not be used simultaneously. Injections should be spaced out within each area, moving one finger-breadth from the previous site:
  - thighs (anterior or lateral) have a slow absorption speed and are suitable for intermediate-acting insulin;
  - the abdomen (the whole of the anterior abdominal wall) has a fast absorption speed and is suitable if fast-acting absorption is required;
  - arms (upper external quadrant) have a medium-to-fast absorption and require shorter needles.

Table 7.5. Choosing the appropriate needle size and injection technique[20]

Patient	Injection technique	Needle size (mm)
Overweight adult	Pinch-up, 90° No pinch-up, 45° No pinch-up	12.7 12.7 8
Normal-weight adult	Pinch-up, 90°	8
Thin adult	No pinch-up, 90°	5 or 6
Children, adolescents	No pinch-up, 90°	5 or 6

    - buttocks (upper outer quadrants) have slow absorption.
- Technique:
  - pinching up the skin (between flexed thumb and index or middle finger) when the injection is given at 90°;
  - choose the right needle size (*Table 7.5*);
  - avoid insulin leakage by waiting 5–10 seconds after the injection to withdraw the needle, doing so as pinch-up is released;
  - inject usually 20–30 minutes before eating, but rapid-acting insulin should be injected just before a meal;
  - good hygiene of site, hands and equipment is essential.

Other points
- Clear instructions about diet are essential and suitable carbohydrate intake between meals may be necessary to prevent hypoglycaemia.
- Care of equipment, storage, keeping spares, noting expiry dates and *correct disposal of sharps* (using a safe-clipper) *and syringes* according to local council guidelines (e.g., in screw top plastic bottles).
- For driving, the patient must inform the licensing centre [Driver and Vehicle Licensing Agency (DVLA)] and driving insurance company.
- Patients should be taught to recognise the causes and features of hypoglycaemia. They should be advised to carry both treatment (glucose sweets or fruit drink followed by longer-acting carbohydrates) and identification (card, necklace or bracelet) at all times.

Possible future developments in blood glucose lowering treatment

In addition to the new approaches discussed below, fixed-dose combinations of established oral blood glucose lowering agents may return to favour and become available in the UK, if only to improve compliance by reducing the number of tablets patients have to swallow. An example is the combination of glibenclamide and metformin, currently available in the USA.

Improving insulin release
A number of new approaches with the potential to enhance insulin secretion are being explored currently.[5] These include:
- The intestinal hormone *glucagon-like peptide-1* (GLP-1) that potentiates nutrient-stimulated insulin secretion (synchronising insulin secretion with food consumption);
- *Succinate esters* targeted at beta cells to stimulate proinsulin biosynthesis and insulin secretion by enhancing the Krebs cycle;
- *Imidazoline compounds*;
- *Phosphodiesterase inhibitors* targeted at beta cells, which might promote insulin secretion by other agents.

Improving insulin action
Potential future therapies for reducing insulin resistance include:
- Newer glitazones or PPAR-γ agonists.

- Vanadium salts reduce hepatic glucose production and enhance insulin-mediated glucose use in muscle by inhibiting (at least in part) the deactivation of insulin receptors. However, any agent that comes into use will need to overcome the risk of vanadium accumulation, which is toxic.
- Substances that enhance insulin-receptor signalling by phosphatase inhibition may have potential, if found.
- Other agents that may have potential are magnesium salts or chromium, for those people deficient in these minerals, and pramlintide, an injectable peptide that reduces weight gain by delayed gastric emptying and satiety.

Alternative insulin delivery systems

In view of many diabetics' distaste for and fear of injections, scientists have been seeking alternative ways for patients to receive insulin. Two promising areas are:

- Different routes of insulin administration (e.g., via nasal mucous membranes or via inhalation); and
- Transplantation of donor islet cells that would then produce insulin in response to blood glucose levels, but preventing rejection requires expensive medication that has its own side effects.

Special Circumstances

Ramadan

During Ramadan, the ninth lunar month in the Islamic calendar year, fasting (no food or drink) between dawn and sunset is obligatory for all healthy Moslem adults. Although certain groups, including ill people, are exempt from fasting, many patients with diabetes may choose to fast and could seek medical advice.[21] It is worth knowing if patients have had previous experience of fasting and whether they are prepared to break the fast if hypoglycaemia occurs.

Diet

There is a major change in the dietary pattern. There are usually two meals, one when the day's fast has finished and one before the next fast begins (this may be at a very early hour). Large quantities of sugary fluids, carbohydrate-rich meals and fried foods may be consumed. Patients may be advised to reduce their intake of these items.

Oral medication

Metformin should be taken at the end of fast to cover the period of eating, but consider reducing the dose or stopping if the patient feels unwell. If on a sulphonylurea, consider changing to a quicker-acting one, such as tolbutamide or glipizide, to be taken once daily before the break-of-fast meal. Repaglinide is a useful alternative when fasting because of its short duration of action.

Insulin

Consider advising a reduction of dose and an avoidance of pre-mixed insulin during fasting. A suitable regimen may be isophane only before the early morning start of the fast meal, and mainly *short*, possibly with a small dose of isophane before the evening break-of-fast meal.

Key Points in this Chapter

- Achieving and maintaining optimal glycaemic control requires the balancing and self-monitoring of diet, physical activity and blood glucose lowering medication.

- Self-monitoring, preferably with plasma glucose, enables patients to adjust their treatment.

- The optimal diet in diabetics should provide essential nutrition, reduce vascular risk and adapt to metabolic problems. Food intake must be balanced with exercise and hypoglycaemic treatment (drugs or insulin), so as to avoid hypoglycaemia and hyperglycaemia.

- Less than 10% of energy intake should be from saturated fats and the total amount of carbohydrate seems to be more important than the source or type.

- The choice of treatment should follow a 'step-up' policy, in the knowledge that pancreatic beta cell function will deteriorate over time, and so result in most type 2 diabetics eventually requiring insulin to achieve acceptable glycaemic control. The combination of the self-monitoring of results, a recent glycated haemoglobin and the patient's well-being should guide both dose changes and decisions about additional medication (or a step-up).

- Conversion to insulin in primary care can be successful if proper training (of both patient and professional) occurs and a suitable insulin regimen is chosen.

REFERENCES

1 Duncan C (Ed.) *Monthly Index of Medical Specialities.* London: Haymarket Medical Publishing, 2003 (updated monthly).

2 Rohlfing CL, Wiedmeyer HM, Little RR *et al.* Defining the relationship between plasma gkucose and HbA1c analysis of glucose profiles and HbA1c in the Diabetes Control and Complications Trial. *Diabetes Care* 2002; 25; 275–278.

3 Toeller M. Diet and diabetes. In: *Diabetes Med.*, 27: 15–18.

4 Leicestershire Health. *Dietary Recommendations for Adults with Diabetes in Leicestershire.* Leicester: Leicestershire Health, 1997.

5 Krentz AJ, Bailey CJ. *Type 2 Diabetes in Practice.* London: Royal Society of Medicine Press Limited, 2001.

6 American Diabetes Association Position Statement. Evidence-based nutrition principles and recommendations for the treatment and prevention of diabetes and related complications. *Diabetes Care* 2003; 26(Suppl. 1): S51–S61.

6 Christiansen C, Thomsen C, Rasmussen O, *et al.* The acute impact of ethanol on glucose, insulin, triacylglycerol, and free fatty acid responses and insulin sensitivity in type 2 diabetes. *Br J Nutr* 1996; 22: 669–675.

8 Joint Formulary Committee. *British National Formulary 44.* London: British Medical Association and

Royal Pharmaceutical Society of Great Britain, 2002.

9 NICE Guideline Development Group and Recommendations Panel. *Inherited Clinical Guideline G. Management of type 2 diabetes: Management of blood glucose.* London: NHS National Institute for Clinical Excellence, 2002. Online: http://www.nice.org.uk

10 Salpeter S, Greyber F, Pasternak G, *et al.* Risk of nonfatal lactic acidosis with metformin use in type 2 diabetes mellitus. *Cochrane Database Syst Rev* 2002; 2: CD002967.

11 Jones GC, Macklin JP, Alexander WD. Contraindications to the use of metformin (Editorial). *BMJ* 2003; 326: 4–5.

12 Krentz AJ, Bailey CJ, Melander A. Thiazolidinediones for type 2 diabetes (Editorial). *BMJ* 2000; 321: 252–253.

13 Day C. Thiazolidinediones: a new class of antidiabetic drugs. *Diabet Med* 1999; 16: 179–192.

14 NICE Appraisal Committee. *Technology Appraisal Guidance No. 9: Guidance on rosiglitazone for type 2 diabetes.* London: NHS National Institute for Clinical Excellence, 2000. Online: http://www.nice.org.uk

15 NICE Appraisal Committee. *Technology Appraisal Guidance No. 21: Guidance on pioglitazone for type 2 diabetes.* London: NHS National Institute for Clinical Excellence, 2001. Online: http://www.nice.org.uk

16 American Diabetes Association. Clinical Practice Recommendations, Position statement: Insulin

administration. *Diabetes Care* 2003; 26 (Suppl. 1): S121–S124.

17 NICE Appraisal Committee. Technology Guidance Appraisal No. 53: Guidance on the use of long-acting insulin analogues for the treatment of diabetes – insulin glargine. London: National Institute for Clinical Excellence, 2002. Online: http://www.nice.org.uk

18 Personal communication from Sister Elaine Curley at the East Leicester Medical Practice.

19 Avery L, Moore S. Changing from tablets to insulin (Fact Sheet 13). *Diabetes Update* 1999.

20 Wilbourne J. Administration of insulin by injection. *Practical Diabetes Int* 2002; 19: S1–S4.

21 Burden ML, Burden AC. *Guidelines for Ramadan in the Diabetic Population*. Leicester: University Hospitals of Leicester Trust, 2000.

CHAPTER EIGHT

Periodic Review

General Considerations

NSF
4
10
11
12

Rationale

The periodic review is at the centre of structured diabetic care. When undertaken regularly, it facilitates collaboration between each diabetic and the involved health care professional(s) with the objectives of:

- Optimising glycaemic control;
- Optimising lifestyle and quality of life;
- Modifying risk factors for vascular disease;
- Identifying and minimising the effect of diabetic complications.

How often should a periodic review be undertaken?

Expert consensus and logistical considerations suggest that a full periodic review should be undertaken once annually. However, some components (particularly glycated haemoglobin and blood pressure) may require more frequent evaluation, both to achieve and to remain on target. A sensible compromise might be to undertake an interim review, every 4–6 months, of glycated haemoglobin, blood pressure and any other components that may require intervention. The organisation of the periodic review is discussed in Chapter 5.

Selecting what to check

It is possible to compile an extensive list of components to be checked for each diabetic during the full periodic review. However, a practice team is more likely to achieve the aims of diabetic care stated at the beginning of this and Chapter 5 if it concentrates on performing the 'essential' checks to the highest possible standard in the widest possible number of patients with diabetes.

Therefore, selection of the 'essential' components required in all periodic reviews should be based upon sound evidence to justify their inclusion (starting with the NSF and NICE official guidance), and upon the capacity of the team to undertake them to a high satisfactory standard. Practices may wish to incorporate additional checks into their periodic review protocols. It is essential that practices should be prepared to review regularly the selection of components in their protocols (as well as targets and interventions), as new evidence and expert advice become available.

In *Table 8.1*, the author's suggested list of components for regular review consists of four sections, each linked to one of the objectives of the review, and subdivided into components, nineteen in total. Some components may be relevant to more than one section (e.g., diet for both glycaemic control and lifestyle.

Table 8.1. A suggested list of the 'essential' components to check in all type 2 diabetics

Section	Components
Assessment of glycaemic control	Symptoms of hyperglycaemia and/or hypoglycaemia Self-monitoring results Glycated haemoglobin
Life style and risk factors	Diet Exercise and physical activity Smoking Blood pressure Weight (including BMI) Serum lipids
Complications	Feet Eyes Albuminuria Serum creatinine Neuropathy Erectile dysfunction (if male) Injection sites (if on insulin)
Administrative	Medication review Date of next follow-up Data entry

The recommendations herein should be implemented according to the individual patient's clinical status and other circumstances. Making good decisions about management in partnership with patients requires a full awareness of all the other factors that affect their lives. There may be occasions when these other factors may assume greater importance to patients than their diabetes.

The National Clinical Guidelines for type 2 diabetes recommend an annual estimate of coronary heart risk for all people without manifest cardiovascular disease (CVD).[1] The list of components for the full periodic review given in *Table 8.1* enables this assessment (and a calculated estimate for the 10-year coronary event risk – see Chapter 9) to take place.

How useful are targets?

The rationale for aggressive treatment of raised blood glucose, dyslipidaemia and hypertension has been made on usually sound scientific evidence and has been accepted by the guiding bodies. The Diabetes NSF and other expert bodies have or will set targets for many of the metabolic and vascular components listed in *Table 8.1* and discussed in this chapter. The quality of care delivered by a health care system will be measured increasingly by how frequently the targets are met.

However, targets that are endpoints do not reflect the amount of change. Also, targets should be achievable or realistic in patients with diabetes. In high-risk patients, intervention should aim to change all reversible risk factors.[2] A more detailed discussion of the evaluation of overall risk and setting targets is given in Chapter 9.

Discussion of the components of the periodic check in this chapter

The discussion is divided into the following subsections, which may overlap between components:

- Rationale;
- Target(s);
- Who assesses;
- Evaluation; and
- Intervention.

Starting the Periodic Review

Effective consultation techniques (see Chapter 12 for further discussion) should be used in the diabetic review, as in all patient encounters. Before launching into the review, it is important for the health care professional to settle the patient and ensure that each patient has an opportunity to raise any concerns. Professionals should remember that patients are the managers of their disease and that any changes in patients' behaviour can only occur if they are willing and able. A suitable greeting can be open ended and friendly, such as, 'How are you getting on?' To ensure that each patient's agenda is not missed, a question along the lines of 'Is there anything that I need to do or remember today?' is helpful. Any cues picked up at the outset or during the review need to be followed up at some point and this needs to be apparent to the patient, otherwise the patient may have the impression of not being listened to.

Although the main agenda of the consultation is the diabetic review, the professional needs to maintain a broader perspective. Psychological and other health problems may be present. Their presence may affect the process of diabetic care. If the review is not the most suitable setting to tackle additional problems, the professional should ensure that an appropriate follow-up is arranged.

Glycaemic Control

Overview

Poor glycaemic control causes the patient to feel less well and increases the risk of complications. The professional needs to collate information from a variety of sources before negotiating a plan of action with the patient.

Assessment of symptoms of hyperglycaemia and hypoglycaemia

Rationale

Hyperglycaemia is not always symptomatic in type 2 diabetics, and its onset can be gradual. Specific questions may be required and the responses could provide cues for other areas to consider. Hypoglycaemia is dangerous.

Target

The target is to ascertain if either hyperglycaemia or hypoglycaemia is present.

Who assesses?

The GP or practice nurse makes the assessment.

Evaluation

The patient should be asked:

- About the presence of hyperglycaemia symptoms and their duration – polyuria followed by polydipsia and weight loss, blurred vision, fatigue, nausea, recurrent infections (e.g., thrush);
- About the nature, frequency and timing of any hypoglycaemic episodes;
- If on insulin or sulphonylureas, are a diabetic card and 'instant' glucose routinely carried?

Intervention

The main intervention is educational: the patient needs to be confident about identifying symptoms and the action to take. Further discussions of diet and treatment are given in Chapter 7, and of exercise later in this chapter.

Patients who do not routinely carry a diabetic card and 'instant' glucose should be advised to do so. Prescribing glucagon may be appropriate for patients with recurrent severe hypoglycaemia. If this is done, the prescriber should ensure that whoever (patient or others) administers the injection is competent and that the current supply remains within the expiry date.

Self-monitoring results

For further discussion of self-monitoring, see Chapter 7 also.

Rationale

Since the symptoms of hyperglycaemia can be moderate or absent, inspection of the patient's own results can give the professional not only information about the fluctuations of plasma glucose, but also valuable information about the patient's knowledge (interpretation of results), skills (testing technique) and attitudes towards the disease. This is particularly important if there is recurrent hypoglycaemia or other evidence of poor glycaemic control. However, self-monitoring should be taught only if the need and/or purpose is clear and agreed with the patient.[3]

Target

To ensure an accurate technique is used and the correct interpretation of tests.

Who assesses?

The GP or practice nurse makes the assessment.

Evaluation

Ideally, the patients should bring their results to the review. The first consideration is whether the timing and frequency of testing provides the patients with sufficient information to control their plasma glucose adequately.

Bear in mind the HbA1c (see next section) when studying self-monitoring results. If there is an incongruity between the overall trend of self-monitoring and the concurrent HbA1c, it may be worthwhile to:

- Observe the patient doing the test – is it carried out and interpreted correctly?
- Ascertain that any blood glucose machine being used is calibrated, and check the strips used are correct and in date.
- Check if the patient records the findings correctly in a retrievable form.

The computerised repeat prescribing record, as part of the medication review (see later), often gives useful information about compliance and usage of prescribed treatment.

Intervention
Encourage the patients to record systematically their results. If urine testing does not provide adequate information, consider asking and teaching the patients how to test their blood. If blood testing, ensure that the patients are prescribed the correct type and sufficient quantity of test strips and lancets.

Glycated haemoglobin

Rationale
Glycated haemoglobin (HbA1c) is formed by nonenzyme glycation (implicated in the pathogenesis of long-term diabetic complications, see Chapter 3) of part of the β-chain of red cell haemoglobin. The proportion of HbA1c to total haemoglobin (as a percentage) is a useful index of *average* blood glucose levels over the preceding 6–8 weeks. There is a correlation between Hb1Ac and the mean plasma glucose; an HbA1c of 7% correlates with a mean glucose level of 9.5mmol/l, rising by 2mmol/l for each 1% increase of HbA1c (see Appendix 1).[4] The UKPDS demonstrated that very good glycaemic control (an average HbA1c of 7.0%) significantly reduced the risk both of microvascular complications (e.g., retinopathy, nephropathy) and of macrovascular disease (e.g., CHD, major stroke) in patients with type 2 diabetes.[5] The progressive deterioration of pancreatic insulin secretion in the disease process and the tight targets for HbA1c require regular estimation, with a frequency of at least twice per year.

Target
The ideal is to achieve an HbA1c as low as possible, while avoiding hypoglycaemia. An HbA1c of less than 6% demonstrates very good control (values may vary slightly in different laboratories). The recommended HbA1c target for optimal glycaemic control varies slightly between different expert groups:

* NICE's Clinical Guideline published in 2002 recommends that an individualised HbA1c target should be set between 6.5 and 7.5%, with the lower target preferred for patients at significant risk of vascular complications, but the higher target for those at risk of iatrogenic hypoglycaemia.[3]
* The European Diabetes Policy Group's recommended target is 6.5% or less.[6]
* The ADA's recommended target is 7.0% or less.[7]

Less strict targets may be appropriate in elderly patients with a limited life expectancy. Also, in view of the progressive deterioration of pancreatic insulin secretion in the disease process, to achieve an HbA1c of 6.5–7.0% or less becomes more difficult and less likely as the duration of diabetes increases. Setting an individualised target, as recommended by Winocour,[8] may be the most pragmatic solution.

Who assesses?
The GP or practice nurse makes the assessment.

Evaluation
NICE recommends that the glycated haemoglobin assay should be aligned with the HbA1c assay used in the DCCT and UKPDS. Most UK hospital laboratories now align their assays accordingly. If a practice acquires a machine for near-patient estimation of HbA1c, it too should be so aligned. It is essential that the results be available at the periodic reviews.

Intervention

- If HbA1c is less than the target, reinforce the patient's good practices and repeat in 6 months.
- If HbA1c is within 1% above the target, consider a review of the diet and exercise levels, and consider a readjustment of the medication (either increase the dose of current drugs or step-up as in *Table 6.3*). HbA1c should be repeated at 3–4 months.
- If HbA1c is more than 1% above the target, a major review of diet, exercise levels and medication is necessary. If the patient is on the near or maximal dose of oral drugs, serious consideration should be given to introducing insulin. HbA1c should be repeated at 2–3 months.
- If unable to achieve satisfactory control despite the above measures, referral to a diabetes specialist nurse or to a hospital diabetic clinic is recommended.

To achieve a target of 7.0% requires many (at least 50%?) patients with type 2 diabetes to be treated with insulin, which has significant 'resource implications' (i.e., costs the country a lot of money) and may not be acceptable or entirely beneficial to many obese patients. Also, intensive treatment to control blood glucose increases the risk of hypoglycaemia.[9]

Lifestyle and Risk Factors

Diet

Fuller discussions of dietary recommendations are given in Chapter 7, of health education in Chapter 12 and of exercise and weight in later sections in this chapter.

Rationale

Healthy eating is an essential component of diabetes health care and behaviour. Knowing and following a suitable diet has a beneficial effect on weight, metabolic control and well being. Healthy eating can contribute to a lowering of vascular risk by reducing central obesity, improving the serum lipid profile and lowering blood pressure, all of which are more dangerous in patients with diabetes.[10]

Target

The target should be to ensure that the patient knows and is following an optimal diet with the following aims (as stated in Chapter 7):

- Provision of essential nutrition;
- Reduction of the risk of vascular complications;
- Adaptation to metabolic problems (food intake must be balanced with exercise and hypoglycaemic treatment, to avoid either hypoglycaemia or hyperglycaemia).

Who assesses?

The practice nurse, dietician and/or the GP make the assessment.

Evaluation

A dietary history helps to assess intake, knowledge and attitude to change (using the trans-theoretical model of change discussed in Chapter 12). This needs to be combined with information about glycaemic control, weight and exercise. The professional also needs to be aware of any relevant social or cultural factors.

Intervention

Both attitude to change and social and/or cultural factors influence the aims and nature of any intervention. Approaches to changing behaviour are discussed in Chapter 12.

Referral to a dietician is indicated if the specific circumstances require more expert assessment and education. If significant changes are recommended, an earlier review is indicated to assess progress.

Dietary recommendations are discussed in detail in Chapter 7. Dietary advice must be realistic and compatible with the advice offered on treatment and exercise. Numerous examples of written advice are available. In Leicestershire the dietetic service has agreed the advice it gives to diabetic patients, as listed in *Table 8.2*.

'Dietary failure' is evident when an overweight patient gains further weight, the likely result of noncompliance with dietary advice. Noncompliance can be caused by:

- Failure to persuade the patient into a stage of being willing and then prepared to change;
- Inadequate assessment of the patient's current diet, cultural or religious customs;
- Poor explanation of the rationale of dietary changes;
- Prescription of a diet that is unpalatable, not satisfying or too expensive;
- Unrealistic expectations and disappointment about the rate of weight loss;
- Craving for sweets or overeating at the same time as trying to stop smoking.

The management of noncompliance is difficult and not often very successful. Direct confrontation is unhelpful and damages the future relationship with the patient. Strategies that involve simplifying advice, building on positive steps already taken by the patient and drawing up a 'contract' with rewards are more likely to produce improvement. If these measures fail, particularly in a very obese type 2 patient, it may be helpful to seek specialist help. Strategies that involve very low calorie diets (VLCDs), anti-obesity drugs and surgical intervention are not without risk, and few GPs or practice nurses have sufficient experience to advise and support patients fully.

Exercise and physical activity

Physical activity is defined as any skeletal muscle movement that expends energy above resting level. Exercise is a type of physical activity that is carried out to enhance or maintain an aspect of fitness.

NSF
1

Table 8.2. Leicestershire guidelines for healthy eating[11]

Eat regular meals and snacks as necessary (eat a variety of different foods)
Eat more high-fibre carbohydrate (starchy) foods
Eat less sugar and avoid sugary foods (do not add sugar to drinks or cereals)
Cut down on the amount of fat and fatty food eaten (e.g., fried foods)
Eat more fruit and vegetables
Avoid special diabetic products (they are expensive and usually high in fat)
Avoid being overweight
If you enjoy a drink (a word of caution), consume alcohol in moderation

Rationale

The underlying message is that 'the correct type of exercise is good'. Exercise has both short- and long-term benefits in type 2 patients (*Table 8.3*). Exercise can be an effective way to reduce the risk of CVD,[12] which is the most common cause of death in type 2 diabetics (see Chapter 3). An appropriate level of physical activity, particularly in conjunction with diet, can improve other vascular risk factors, such as blood pressure, weight and lipids.

Targets

To undertake regular *enjoyable* physical activity that will promote endurance, muscle strength and flexibility, and reduce cardiovascular risk (also see below).

Who assesses?

The practice nurse, GP and exercise physiologist (if available) make the assessment.

Evaluation

Evaluation may be difficult. As well as eliciting details about the frequency, duration, type and intensity of physical activity, the professional should consider the attitude of the patient towards exercise, and social and cultural factors.

Prior to beginning an exercise programme, diabetics need to be screened for the following:

* *Peripheral neuropathy* may result in loss of protective sensation in the feet. Therefore, repetitive exercise can be traumatic to insensitive feet and ultimately can lead to ulceration and fractures. Treadmill, jogging and step exercises are not suitable in these patients, whereas nonweight-bearing exercises, such as swimming, cycling and arm-and-chair exercises, avoid this risk. Proper footwear and adequate foot care are always necessary (see *Table 8.13*).

Table 8.3. The benefits of exercise for type 2 patients[13,14]

Metabolic:
* reduced short-term insulin resistance; long-term effect has yet to be established
* increased peripheral glucose uptake
* less atherogenic profile (decreased triglycerides and LDL cholesterol with a beneficial increase in HDL cholesterol)
* there is still no clear consensus on whether physical training results in improved fibrinolytic activity, which is impaired in type 2 diabetics

Reduces hypertension, a known cardiovascular risk factor

Helps to maintain muscle mass and promote preferentially the loss of adipose tissue, which may reduce the fall in metabolic rate during slimming and accelerate long-term weight loss

Favours weight loss by increasing energy expenditure (although an ageing overweight type 2 diabetic will be hard pressed to maintain the necessary daily level of exercise), but is best combined with a slimming diet

Prevention: physical activity undertaken in early adult life protects against the subsequent development of type 2 diabetes in middle-aged men and women[15] and in patients with impaired glucose tolerance[16]

- Patients with *active retinopathy,* in particular *proliferative*, must avoid activities that increase systolic blood pressure, involve Valsalva manoeuvres or are jarring, since these can increase substantially the risk of retinal detachment.[17]
- Patients with known *coronary artery disease* require proper evaluation of the ischaemic response to exercise and the propensity to arrhythmia during exercise.

Intervention

As with dietary advice, both attitude to change and social and/or cultural factors need to be considered before undertaking any exercise programme (see Chapter 12). The goals set by the patient and professional determine the balance, duration, intensity and methods of exercise to undertake after the evaluation. Ideally, a complete exercise programme combines aerobic (e.g., walking, running, cycling, dancing, swimming, skipping) and anaerobic (e.g., resistive strength training of major muscle groups) activities. The latter have been shown to reduce vascular risk by decreasing resting blood pressure, increasing HDL cholesterol (HDL-C, see below) and decreasing insulin resistance.

Increasing numbers of practices across the country now can refer suitable patients to exercise programmes run locally, called 'exercise on prescription'. However, health care professionals must take great care to ensure that any exercise programme is safe, appropriate to patients' general physical condition, suitable to their lifestyle and goals, and enjoyable. As with nondiabetic patients, it is important that exercise includes proper warm-up and cooldown periods; this should also reduce the risk of injury.

The 'ideal' is set out in *Table 8.4*, but this may not be desirable or realistic for all patients with diabetes.

Advice is needed to help diabetics to maintain normoglycaemia during exercise (*Table 8.5*).

Smoking

Rationale

Cigarette smoking is a major alterable risk factor in vascular disease, which is closely associated with type 2 diabetes. The UKPDS identified smoking as a risk factor for coronary artery disease in type 2 diabetics.[19] Smoking also promotes the development of microvascular complications of diabetes (retinopathy, nephropathy and foot disease). If patients with diabetes stop smoking, stroke could be reduced by 5%, CHD by 10% and peripheral vascular disease by 30%.[20] The author's limited personal experience of using cardiac risk calculators (see Chapter 9) supports the above-named benefits of smoking cessation.

Targets

The targets are to:

- Elicit if and how much the patient smokes;
- Promote and maintain cessation of smoking.

Who assesses?

The GP or practice nurse makes the assessment.

Evaluation

Patients are asked if and how much they smoke. If a smoker, the patients' willingness to change and any barriers to change need to be established.

Intervention

The patient's position on the trans-theoretical model of change[21] is likely to determine the possible success of any intervention (see further discussion in Chapter 12). If a patient appears unwilling to change, emphasise the positive health and social benefits of becoming a nonsmoker while underlining the considerable risks of remaining a smoker, this attitude may change.

The Cochrane Library (see also Chapter 14) evaluated the evidence for the efficacy of various interventions to promote smoking cessation and concluded that a variety of effective strategies are available.[22] Both nicotine replacement therapy (NRT) and bupropion have been the subjects of NICE guidance:[23]

- If the patient is motivated to stop, the best initial approach is to reinforce the above message and to advise the patient to set a date for stopping. Brief (3 minutes) advice to stop smoking given by a health professional has been shown to reduce the proportion of people who smoke by 2%, compared to providing no advice.[24]
- When combined with NRT, this is doubled in motivated 'quitters' who smoke more than 10 cigarettes per day.[25] NRT is available (as transdermal patches, chewing gum, inhalation or nasal spray) for physical withdrawal symptoms (e.g., first cigarette before breakfast; see BNF Section 4.10 for details[26]). All forms are effective and are available over the counter or on NHS prescription. The dose depends upon the number of cigarettes smoked per day. NRT is fairly safe, but NICE recommends caution in patients with CVD, hyperthyroidism, diabetes, severe renal or hepatic impairment and peptic ulcer.[23] NICE recommends that the initial prescription of NRT should be sufficient to last 2 weeks after the target stop date.[23] Second prescriptions for NRT and bupropion (see below) should only be given to people who have demonstrated that their attempt to quit is still being sustained when reassessed.
- Many health authorities now provide *smoking cessation clinics*, organised within the framework of initiatives such as Health Action Zones (HAZs). Freely accessible and run by trained counsellors, these are more effective than brief advice or usual care in motivated 'quitters'.
- The *antidepressants* bupropion (Zyban; see BNF Section 4.10[26]) and nortriptyline have shown increased cessation rates in a small number of trials, whether or not depression was present. Since patients in these trials were offered behavioural support also, the most logical use of these drugs is in combination with a structured counselling programme.[22] Bupropion is available currently on the NHS. NICE recommends that the initial prescription of bupropion should be sufficient for 3–4 weeks after the target stop date.[23] The main adverse events associated with bupropion are seizures, which occur in about 1 in 1000 patients. In addition, it is also recommended that patients who are prescribed bupropion should have their blood pressure monitored, as rises have been reported, even in normotensive individuals. Both NRT and bupropion should not be prescribed to smokers under the age of 18 years or in combination. NICE recommends that the NHS should not normally fund further treatment with NRT or bupropion within 6 months of a previous unsuccessful attempt using these agents.[23]
- Other methods are either ineffective (anxiolytics and lobeline), of uncertain benefit (acupuncture, aversion therapy, hypnotherapy) or limited by side effects (clonidine).

Blood pressure

For a discussion of blood pressure, also see the recently published National Clinical Guidelines for type 2 diabetes.[27]

Rationale

There is a close association between type 2 diabetes and hypertension, with hypertension appearing to act synergistically to accelerate the development of vascular disease in diabetic patients. The optimal blood pressure for all patients with type 2 diabetics is not known. The UKPDS has shown that lowering blood pressure in patients with type 2 diabetes reduces the risk of deaths related to diabetes, and both microvascular (nephropathy, retinopathy) and macrovascular (e.g., CHD, major stroke) complications related to diabetes.[28]

Target

Neither research evidence nor expert consensus has found a level of blood pressure below which treatment does not confer benefit. Successive sets of guidelines seem to 'compete' for the lowest target blood pressure. The UKPDS and the National Clinical Guidelines for type 2 diabetes have set 140/80mmHg as a target, but recently the ADA recommended a target of less than 130/80mmHg.[29] Whatever target is used, a lower level seems sensible if target organ damage is present. Less strict targets may be appropriate in elderly patients with limited life expectancy. As discussed at the start of this chapter, to achieve such tight targets may not be possible in or acceptable to some patients with type 2 diabetes, despite or because of the concurrent prescribing of several agents. It should not be forgotten that any lowering of blood pressure reduces vascular risk in any patient with diabetes (see Chapter 9): most of the cited studies achieved reductions of the order of 10/5mmHg. Thus, rather than aiming invariably for a fixed endpoint, an individualised target based upon the starting level of blood pressure and an achievable reduction may be more realistic and appropriate.

Who assesses?

The GP or practice nurse makes the assessment.

Evaluation

Measuring the blood pressure

The patient should be seated or supine, and the cuff bladder size should be a suitable one for the patient's arm (obese arms need a large cuff). It is recommended that blood pressure should be measured in both arms on the first visit. The diastolic pressure is recorded at the disappearance of sound (phase V). If the reading is larger than the targets stated above, further readings need to be taken on separate visits.

A variety of automated sphygmomanometers are now available for professional and self-use. Before purchasing any model, the buyer is advised to enquire whether the device has passed independent validation using the protocols of the British Hypertension Society (BHS) and the Association for the Advancement of Medical Instrumentation Standard (AAMI).[30] Further useful advice may be available from the local hospital's medical physics department. Mercury sphygmomanometers are still legal and they can be as accurate (when set up properly) as the best-automated machine. Many aneroid sphygmomanometers lose accuracy when jolted.

Target organ damage

Any evidence of target organ damage should be sought. The 'organs' to consider are the eyes (retinopathy), kidneys (proteinuria, renal impairment), heart [left ventricular hypertrophy (LVH)] and feet (neuropathy, impaired circulation and/or foot ulcer).

Potential causes of hypertension
If there are any underlying causes of hypertension, is the lifestyle (diet, alcohol, smoking, lack of exercise) a contributory factor? Some types of medication can cause raised blood pressure, such as cold cures, hormone replacement therapy, oral corticosteroids, nonsteroidal anti-inflammatory drugs, and carbenoxolone. Examination occasionally reveals palpable kidneys (which could indicate polycystic kidneys or an adrenal mass), renal bruits (which may indicate renovascular disease) and delayed or absent femoral pulses (which occur in co-arctation of the aorta).

Family history
The family history must be checked for hypertension, vascular or renal disease.

Investigations
For patients with raised blood pressure or when hypertension is diagnosed, investigations are:
- Urea and electrolyte estimation is essential to establish if there is renal impairment (hypokalaemia on no medication occurs in hyperaldosteronism);
- If renal disease or renal artery stenosis is suspected, a renal ultrasound is useful and available to GPs.

Further investigations are best done under specialist supervision.

Interventions
The main aim here is reduce the overall cardiovascular risk.

To treat or not to treat?
A single measurement is rarely sufficient to determine an individual's 'true' blood pressure level and, thus, to justify a decision on whether to treat. Repeated measurements need to be taken over a length of time. The duration of observation prior to a treatment decision depends upon how elevated the blood pressure measurements are, and if target organ damage and/or any other vascular risk factors are present. If the measurements are elevated only slightly and there is no target organ damage in a 'low risk' individual, it is reasonable to observe the patient over several months. If the measurements are elevated markedly or target organ damage is present in a 'higher risk' individual, a briefer duration of observation with earlier intervention is indicated. If there is considerable variation between measurements or if there is the possibility of 'white coat' hypertension, it may prove helpful to organise 24-hour ambulatory blood-pressure monitoring.

Nonpharmacological methods
Nonpharmacological methods are indicated in all patients. As for all diabetic patients, those with raised blood pressure should be urged to not smoke, restrict alcohol, reduce salt intake, take more exercise and eat healthily (see above). It must not be forgotten that good glycaemic control reduces vascular risk.

Pharmacological methods
The huge range and quantity of blood pressure lowering drugs available mirrors that of blood glucose lowering medication. Before discussing the individual drug classes, several key concepts need to be borne in mind:
- *Several factors dictate the first-line choice of drug to be used.* Currently, these include efficacy, whether any diabetic complications and/or cardiovascular risk factors are present, the ethnic origin of the patient, the potential side effects of the drug and the risk of inter-

Table 8.6. National Clinical Guideline recommendations for the pharmacological management of raised blood pressure (mmHg) in people with type 2 diabetes

Step	Blood pressure (BP)	10-year coronary event risk	Microalbuminuria or proteinuria present?	Recommendations*
1	≥140/80 and <160/100	Lower	No	Monitor BP regularly (twice per year) If 10-year risk increases to higher level, treat according to step 2 If BP consistently ≥160/100, treat according to step 3
2	≥140/80 and <160/100	Higher	No	Offer pharmacological treatment (first-line ACE/ARA, beta-blocker or thiazide diuretic) Aim for target BP <140/80
3	≥160/100	Higher or lower	No	Offer pharmacological treatment (first-line ACE/ARA, beta-blocker or thiazide diuretic) Aim for target BP <140/80
4	≥140/80	Higher or lower	Yes	Offer pharmacological treatment Aim for target BP ≤135/75 ACE as first-line if proteinurea or microalbuminuria (use ARA as alternative if ACE unsuitable or contraindicated) In combination with ACE or ARA, can use beta-blocker, long-acting CCB or thiazide diuretic

*ACE, angiotensin-converting enzyme; ARA, angiotensin-II receptor antagonists; CCBs, calcium channel blockers.

action with other medication. In future, the likely greater understanding of the mechanism(s) of raised blood pressure in individuals may give rise to new drug classes or more effective targeting of existing drugs to correct specific defects at the cellular level.

- *Combinations of more than one drug class.* These will be required to gain and maintain adequate blood pressure control in many patients.
- *Actual level of blood pressure achieved.* This may be more important than the class of drug(s) used. The UKPDS showed captopril (an ACE inhibitor) and atenolol (a beta-blocker) to be

equally effective in reducing the incidence of diabetic complication;[31] similarly, the ALLHAT (antihypertensive and lipid lowering to prevent heart attack trial) study found thiazides, ACE inhibitors and calcium channel blocker (CCB) comparable in reducing blood pressure and cardiovascular events.[32]

- *Safety and relative efficacy.* Further evidence is required to remove uncertainty over the safety and relative efficacy of some blood pressure lowering drugs.

Table 8.6 sets out the recently published recommendations made in the National Clinical Guidelines for type 2 diabetes for the pharmacological management of raised blood pressure.[27] For practical purposes, patients are subdivided into *higher* (history of CVD or 10-year coronary event risk of >15%) and *lower* (no CVD history and 10-year risk of ≤15%) coronary event risk (set out in *Table 9.1*). However, the author believes that this guidance, particularly in step 1, is not entirely logical or clearly set out for the following reasons:

- All type 2 diabetics should be considered at high risk of developing CVD (see the discussions in Chapters 3 and 9) over their lifetimes.
- Not to recommend pharmacological treatment of blood pressure levels between 140/80 and 160/100mmHg in a substantial proportion of patients with type 2 diabetes is inconsistent with other current authoritative guidance,[29] the National Clinical Guidelines' own stated target blood pressure of 140/80mmHg and the results of various landmark studies, such as the UKPDS.[28]

The main drug classes that can be used to treat raised blood pressure in diabetics are ACE inhibitors or angiotensin-II receptor antagonists (ARA), beta-blockers, thiazide diuretics, long-acting CCBs, alpha 1 adrenergic blockers and centrally acting antihypertensive agents. The most recent guidance from the ADA recommends initial drug therapy 'with any drug class currently indicated for the treatment of hypertension', with 'some drug classes (ACE inhibitors, beta-blockers and thiazide diuretics) shown to be particularly beneficial in reducing CHD events ... and, therefore, preferred agents for initial therapy'.[29]

Both *ACE inhibitors and ARAs* inhibit the rennin–angiotensin system. Both classes conserve renal function in diabetic nephropathy and are beneficial in heart failure, although currently only ACE inhibitors have a UK licence for the treatment of heart failure. ACE inhibitors (with ARA as an alternative) are the recommended first-line class of drugs to be prescribed in patients with both raised blood pressure and microalbuminuria or proteinuria (see *Table 8.6*).

The older class is the ACE inhibitors (the many examples include captopril, enalapril, lisinopril, perindopril, quinapril, ramipril, trandolapril – all generic names end in 'pril'; see BNF Section 2.5.5.1 for doses[26]). The HOPE study reported that treatment using ramipril in a 'high risk' group of men aged at least 55 years with a history of CHD, stroke, peripheral vascular disease or diabetes, and an additional cardiovascular risk factor, reduced the risk of stroke and of myocardial infarction, independently of reduction in blood pressure.[33] It is not entirely clear whether this was because of a specific effect of ramipril itself or because of ACE inhibitors as a class. Currently, NICE is conducting a technology appraisal of ramipril and other ACE inhibitors.

ARAs (e.g., candesartan, irbesartan, losartan, telmisartan, valsartan – all generic names end in 'sartan'; see BNF Section 2.5.5.2 for doses[26]) have been introduced recently and do not have the side effect of cough that the ACE inhibitors have. The LIFE study concluded that cardiovascular morbidity and death in hypertensive patients with electrocardiographic evidence of LVH, especially the study's diabetic subgroup, was reduced by treatment with the ARA losartan.[34] As in the HOPE study, there is some controversy about the interpretation and significance of the findings, and extrapolation of LIFE's findings to hypertensive patients without LVH should be resisted until further supporting evidence is published.

Both ACE inhibitors and ARAs should be used only with caution (and perhaps after seeking specialist advice) in patients with peripheral vascular disease, renovascular disease and a raised serum creatinine (>120nmol/l). Thus, the serum potassium and creatinine should be checked prior to and within 7–10 days of starting treatment and after each increase in dose, as a rise might indicate renal damage (possibly through renal artery stenosis) that is irreversible if the drug is not stopped. ACE inhibitors have no effect on lipid metabolism or glucose tolerance, but are less effective in Afro-Caribbean patients (ARAs are effective in this ethnic group). The candesartan and lisinopril microalbuminuria (CALM) study suggested that the combination of the ACE inhibitor lisinopril with the ARA candesartan may be more effective in reducing blood pressure and urinary albumin excretion than the individual drugs in type 2 diabetics (although the study dose of lisinopril was only half the maximal dose).[35]

Beta adrenoceptor blocking drugs (many examples, including atenolol, bisoprolol, carvedilol, metoprolol and oxprenolol – all generic names end in 'lol'; see BNF Section 2.4 for doses[26]) are indicated in patients with CHD and in patients with heart failure, but first- and second-generation agents may affect plasma lipids adversely. Beta-blockers may mask hypoglycaemia.

Although *thiazide diuretics* can affect glucose and lipid metabolism adversely (dose-related), they are effective at low dose (e.g., bendrofluazide at 2.5mg in the morning) with minimal adverse metabolic effects. Generic thiazides also have the advantage of being very inexpensive. Recently published results from the ALLHAT study indicate that thiazide-type diuretics are both as effective in reducing blood pressure and cardiovascular events and as well-tolerated as ACE inhibitors and CCBs in patients with hypertension.[32] Long-term use of thiazides can reduce serum sodium and potassium levels, which should be monitored.

CCBs are subdivided into three different classes (see BNF Section 2.6.2 for doses[26]):

* Class I, phenylalkylamines (e.g., verapamil);
* Class II, dihydropyridine CCBs (DCCBs; e.g., amlodipine, nifedipine, lacidipine, felodipine);
* Class III, benzothiazepines (e.g., diltiazem).

Class I agents depress cardiac conduction and may precipitate heart failure if there is AV or SA node dysfunction. Class II agents are relatively selective for the vasculature, and do not depress conduction or contractility, and thus are less likely to precipitate heart failure. Class III agents have a negligible negative inotropic effect and do not cause reflex tachycardia. None of the classes affect plasma lipids or glucose metabolism, and all are effective in Afro-Caribbean patients. There is currently some debate about the efficacy and safety of CCBs. A recent prospective randomised, blinded trial suggested that ACE inhibitors were more effective than CCBs at preventing myocardial infarction in hypertensive patients with diabetes and concerns were raised over the safety of CCBs.[36] The BHS did not support these concerns in their 1999 guidelines.[37] However, at the European Society of Cardiology meeting in August 2000, Furberg and his colleagues presented their meta-analysis of several trials, which suggested no difference in the blood pressure levels achieved by CCBs and non-CCBs, but that patients who received DCCBs were at increased risk of certain major cardiovascular events (is this a question of safety or of efficacy?). Publication of the results from large trials currently in progress should clarify matters. The National Clinical

Guidelines for type 2 diabetes currently recommends the prescription of long-acting (avoid short-acting) CCBs only as second-line treatment or as part of combination therapy.[27]

Alpha 1 adrenergic blockers (e.g., doxazosin, prazosin) are a safe and effective class of drug, and have been shown to improve insulin sensitivity and may improve lipid profiles. They can cause first-dose syncope and orthostatic hypotension, which are best avoided by starting at a low dose and by stopping concomitant diuretics. They are effective in Afro-Caribbean patients.

Centrally acting antihypertensive agents (see Section 2.5.2 of the BNF[26]) include methyl-dopa and moxonidine. The use of these agents should be reserved for patients whose blood pressures have not been controlled by, or in whom there are contraindications to, other blood pressure lowering drugs.

Drug combinations are individual to each patient, and determined by efficacy, tolerability and safety. It is logical to combine drugs from the preferred first-line classes (ACE or ARA, beta-blocker, thiazide), before moving on to second-line classes (CCB, alpha-blocker). Caution is needed if combining a beta-blocker with a DCCB, since this may precipitate heart block or failure.

Blood pressure review
As stated at the start of this chapter, blood pressure is one of the components of the periodic review that should be checked every 4–6 months (at the interim review). If there is an intervention, the interval between blood pressure reviews should be shorter, every 1–3 months, and any side effects monitored.

Referral
Referral is indicated:
- If an underlying cause of hypertension or if an abnormality on physical examination are found;
- If blood pressure control does not achieve its target with the chosen drug(s).

Weight (BMI)
Rationale
Obesity, especially truncal, results in increased insulin resistance and, thus, cardiovascular risk. Reduction of obesity lowers resting blood pressure, and improves lipid profiles and glycaemic control.

Target
The target is a BMI less then 25kg/m^2 in men and 24 kg/m^2 in women, with no central obesity.

Who assesses?
The practice nurse or GP makes the assessment.

Evaluation
The patient should be weighed without shoes, and the height checked if not known, before calculating the BMI.

Intervention
The target weight and rate of loss (ideally 1–2kg/month) should be negotiated, based upon sound health education practice (see Chapter 12). It is sensible to provide simple focused advice about diet and exercise. Earlier review is indicated to monitor progress and to encourage the patient.

Anti-obesity agents may help diabetics to lose weight in combination with a restricted energy diet (and, ideally, increased physical activity). Two main agents are in use, which act by different mechanisms. Neither is cheap and both have been appraised by NICE:

- Orlistat (Xenical) is a long-acting inhibitor of gastrointestinal lipases, and acts within the stomach and small intestine. It works by preventing the hydrolysis and subsequent absorption of ingested dietary fat. It can be prescribed to diabetics aged 18–75 years with a BMI of 28kg/m^2 or more, who can adhere to a hypocaloric diet and who lose at least 2.5kg in weight in the month prior to initiating treatment. The dose is one 120mg capsule with each of the three main meals. Treatment can be continued for up to 12 months (occasionally up to 24 months), provided that a further 5% of body weight is lost by the end of 3 months' treatment and 10% by the end of 6 months.[38] The main side effect is faecal incontinence.
- Sibutramine (Reductil) is an anorectic agent that acts centrally by inhibiting serotonin and noradrenaline reuptake, which results in enhanced satiety. Patients feel satisfied with smaller food portions. Sibutramine has several important contraindications (important macro- and microvascular disease, uncontrolled hypertension, severe renal impairment, glaucoma, benign prostatic hypertrophy with urinary retention) and interacts with other drugs, including antidepressants, and drugs that affect CYP3A4 or serotonin levels. Sibutramine can be prescribed to diabetics aged 18–65 years with a BMI of 27kg/m^2 or more. The starting dose is 10mg daily, but this can be increased to 15mg daily after 4 weeks. Continuation beyond the first 4 weeks requires a weight loss of 2kg, and beyond 3 months a loss of 5% of the initial weight at the start of treatment. The maximum duration of treatment in the licence is 12 months.[39]

Specialist help should be sought if the patient is very obese or fails to respond to intervention.

Serum lipids

Serum lipids are discussed in the recently published National Clinical Guidelines for type 2 diabetes.[40]

Rationale

CHD is the most common cause of morbidity and mortality in type 2 diabetics.[41] Dyslipidaemia (abnormalities of lipids and lipoproteins) occurs often in type 2 patients and is closely related to insulin resistance and hyperinsulinaemia. Increased LDL cholesterol (LDL-C) and triglyceride (TG) levels correlate with, while HDL-C cholesterol levels are inversely related to, the increased risk of developing macrovascular disease.[42] The most common pattern of dyslipidaemia in type 2 diabetics is:

- Elevated TG levels;
- Decreased HDL-C levels;
- Preponderance of LDL-C through lower HDL-C, usually without a significant increase in the absolute concentration of LDL-C.

These lipid abnormalities have been identified by the UKPDS as major risk factors for CHD,[19] but they do respond to intervention. Several large randomised controlled trials, which included type 2 diabetic subjects, have demonstrated reduced CHD incidence and mortality with treatment. Furthermore, the landmark Medical Research Council/British Heart Foundation (MRC/BHF) Heart Protection Study found that treatment of high-risk patients (including diabetics with or without prior CHD) with a high-dose statin reduced the rates of myocardial infarction, stroke and revascularisation by one-quarter, irrespective of the cholesterol level at the start of treatment.[43]

Targets

A logical aim is to both reduce and maintain lipids below the threshold at which the risk of CHD is increased. The National Clinical Guidelines for type 2 diabetes do not recommend treatment if:

- Total cholesterol (TC) is less than 5.0mmol/l (or LDL-C is less than 3.0mmol/l) *and*
- TGs are less than 2.3mmol/l.[40]

These recommendations concur with the Joint British Societies' lipid targets for primary prevention in diabetics (with a 15% or greater risk of developing CHD over the next 10 years; see Chapter 9).[44] The divergence between British and American guidance is now less than previously.

American expert bodies have tended to recommend tougher targets and a more aggressive approach to lipid lowering. The National Cholesterol Education Program proposed that patients with diabetes, irrespective of whether or not CHD is present, should be considered as 'equivalent to' nondiabetic patients with CHD when determining whether lipid-regulating treatment should be given.[45] The most recent position statement published by the ADA recommends the following therapeutic goals:[29]

- LDL-C less than 2.6mmol/l;
- TG less than 1.7mmol/l;
- HDL-C greater than 1.15mmol/l (greater than 1.38mmol/l in women).

However, the recent publication of studies such as the MRC/BHF Heart Protection Study[43] may result in future recommendations (on both sides of the Atlantic) that advise an even more aggressive approach to lipid regulation. Ultimately, one can foresee future guidance with no lower limit for both intervention in and target value of LDL-C in patients with type 2 diabetes.

Less strict targets may be appropriate in some elderly patients with a limited life expectancy.

Who assesses?

The GP or practice nurse makes the assessment.

Evaluation

Serum lipid estimation is best done after an overnight fast, because chylomicrons from the previous meal can affect TG levels. The practice should request that the local chemical pathology laboratory provides TC and lipoprotein fractions, and TG levels. As discussed in Chapter 9, using one of the widely available charts or computer programs to determine the overall cardiovascular risk enables a more accurate assessment of the significance of a given lipid result for each diabetic. However, cardiovascular risk can be underestimated in patients with a positive family history of CHD or in patients from particular ethnic groups. Apart from poor glycaemic control, which contributes to elevated TG levels, lipid levels may be affected by the these nondiabetic factors:

- Genetic disorders, such as familial combined hyperlipidaemia or hypertriglyceridaemia;
- Other diseases, such as hypothyroidism or renal disease;
- Drugs, such as oestrogens;
- Lifestyle, such as alcohol or a diet rich in saturated fat.

Intervention

The primary goal of therapy is to lower LDL-C.

Nonpharmacological

Optimal diet (MNT; see Chapter 7) and increased physical activity (see above) should be attempted, as appropriate, in all patients with dyslipidaemia. Weight loss, reduced alcohol intake and exercise can lead to decreased TG and LDL-C levels, and increased HDL levels. These interventions should be evaluated regularly. Maximal MNT can reduce LDL-C by up to 0.65mmol/l. Unless the patient is at high risk and requires immediate drug treatment, a period of 3–6 months is needed to ascertain if the dietary and/or exercise regime has been successful.

Pharmacological

With the recent National Clinical Guidelines, the previous recommendation of a threshold of a 30% risk of developing a coronary event over 10 years for pharmacological intervention is no longer applicable in type 2 diabetes. A summary of the latest recommendations, based upon the subdivision of 10-year coronary event risk into higher and lower, is set out in *Table 8.7*.[40] As with the blood pressure recommendations, this guidance is neither entirely logical nor clearly set out. To this author, the following makes more sense:

- All type 2 diabetics should be regarded as high risk.
- Why not simply regard initial TC ≥5.0mmol/l and/or LDL-C ≥3.0mmol/l and/or TG ≥2.3mmol/l as requiring treatment and aim to reduce below these targets?
- Irrespective of the initial levels, improving the lipid profile benefits all type 2 diabetics, as supported by the MRC/BHF study cited above.[43]

Several classes of drugs regulate lipids (see BNF Section 2.12 for doses[26]):

- Hydroxymethyl glutaryl coenzyme A (HMG-CoA) reductase inhibitors are commonly known as *statins*. These are more effective in lowering LDL-C than in both reducing TGs and raising HDL-C. The statins currently available in the UK are atorvastatin, fluvastatin, pravastatin and simvastatin. They are currently expensive. Cerivastatin was withdrawn because of the risk of rhabdomyolysis when used in combination with gemfibrozil. Several well-publicised trials demonstrated that pravastatin [CARE (cholesterol and recurrent events[46]), LIPID (long-term intervention with pravastatin in ischaemic disease[47]) and WOSCOPS (West of Scotland coronary prevention study[48])] and simvastatin [4S (Scandinavian simvastatin survival study[49]) and MRC/BHF[43]] reduce both total and LDL-C levels and are effective in the primary and secondary prevention of CHD. A new-generation statin, rosuvastatin, claimed by its manufacturers to be more potent at lowering LDL-C levels, gained regulatory approval in the Netherlands at the end of 2002 and is expected to be approved elsewhere in Europe and in the USA in 2003. This and other 'superstatins' may be referred to NICE for a technology appraisal, because of concerns about costs. Although statins are usually well tolerated, they should be used with caution in patients with a history of liver disease or with a high alcohol intake. Rhabdomyolysis and reversible myositis are rare but significant side effects of statins. Patients should be advised to report promptly unexplained muscle pain, tenderness or weakness. A minority of patients treated with statins do not achieve their lipid-lowering goals.
- *Fibrates* (bezafibrate, ciprofibrate, fenofibrate and gemfibrozil) are broad-spectrum lipid-modulating agents, the main action of which is to decrease serum TG levels. They also tend to reduce LDL-C and to raise HDL-C. Fibrates can cause a myositis-like syndrome, particularly in patients with impaired renal function. Details of doses are found in BNF[26] or MIMS[50].
- *Anion-exchange resins* (cholestyramine and colestipol) reduce LDL-C by binding bile acids, which prevents their reabsorption and so increases LDL-C breakdown. These resins are not especially palatable, can cause gastrointestinal side effects (constipation more than diarrhoea, nausea, vomiting and discomfort) and can aggravate hypertriglyceridaemia.
- *Fish oils* (omega-3-marine TGs) reduce serum TGs.

- *Nicotinic acid group* (nicotinic acid and acipimox) drugs also lower serum TG levels. Of this group, Niacin appears to act in several ways, including partial inhibition of free fatty acid release from adipose tissue, increased lipoprotein lipase activity and decreased hepatic synthesis of LDL-C. An extended-release formulation is available in the USA, as either monotherapy (Niaspan) or fixed combination with lovastatin (Advicor). Both are likely to

Table 8.7. Summary of the National Clinical Guideline's recommendations for lipid-lowering pharmacological therapy*

Blood lipid profile at the start of therapy (mmol/l)	10-year coronary event risk	Recommendations
TC ≥5.0 or LDL-C ≥3.0 or TG >2.3, but <10	Lower (no history of CVD and 10-year coronary event risk ≤15%)	Discuss CHD risk, considering treatment options Consider offering drug therapy at higher TC and TG levels If decided to start treatment, offer statin Monitor treatment 3 monthly and titrate until stable If decision made not to prescribe drugs, monitor lipid profile annually
TC ≥5.0 or LDL-C ≥3.0 or TG >2.3, but <10	Higher (10-year coronary event risk ≥15%, but no CVD history)	Primary prevention: offer a statin; monitor treatment 3 monthly and titrate until stable; monitor lipid profile annually
TC ≥5.0 or LDL-C ≥3.0 or TG >2.3, but <10	Higher (manifest CVD)	Secondary prevention: offer a statin; monitor treatment in 3 months and titrate; consider adding fibrate after 6 months if TG remains ≥2.3; monitor for interaction between statin and fibrate; monitor lipid profile annually
TC <5.0 or LDL-C <3.0 and TG >2.3, but <10	Higher (manifest CVD)	Secondary prevention: offer a statin or a fibrate; monitor treatment 3 monthly and titrate until stable; monitor lipid profile annually
Fasting TG >10	Higher or lower	Offer fibrate therapy Consider referral to specialist clinic

*TC, total cholesterol; TG, triglycerides; CHD, coronary heart disease; CVD, cardiovascular disease.

be introduced soon into Europe. Sustained-release niacin has been associated with cases of severe hepatic toxicity; therefore, niacin should be used with caution in patients with a history of liver disease or who consume large quantities of alcohol.

- *Cholesterol-absorption inhibitors* reduce blood cholesterol by inhibiting absorption of cholesterol by the small intestine. Ezetimibe is the first product in this class and has just gained regulatory approval in the USA and Germany. It is thought that ezetimibe in combination with either a statin or a fibrate could act synergistically to lower LDL-C levels.
- Other pharmacological options include *plant sterols* (no drug preparation, not especially effective) and *antioxidants* (lack of supporting evidence from intervention studies).

Potential cholesterol management agents in development include:

- Avasimibe, an acyl coenzyme A cholesterol acyltransferase (ACAT) inhibitor, is a direct-acting anti-atherosclerotic agent and is in Phase III trials.
- A cholesteryl ester transfer protein (CETP) inhibitor, JTT-705, acts by increasing HDL-C levels and is in Phase II trials.
- A cholesterol vaccine against endogenous CETP may be useful in reducing atherosclerosis risk factors. It, too, is in Phase II trials.

As *Table 8.7* indicates, the choice of drug prescribed depends upon the nature of the dyslipidaemia (not all patients need a statin) and the usual care over tolerability, contraindications and potential interactions.

Once started on treatment, patients require earlier review to monitor the response to and the safety of their treatment. Patients on statins should have liver function tests (LFTs) and creatine kinase (CK) estimations 2–3 months after starting treatment, after any further increase in dose or if symptoms of myositis occur at any time on therapy. The ADA provides a useful guide to the appropriate therapeutic interventions, summarised in *Table 8.8*.

Referral to either a lipid or diabetic clinic is indicated if targets are not achieved or if medication is not tolerated.

Complications

Feet

Feet are also discussed later in the section on Neuropathy.

Rationale

WHO has defined the diabetic foot as a group of syndromes in which neuropathy, ischaemia and infection lead to tissue breakdown, which results in morbidity and possible amputation.[51] Peripheral neuropathy causes lost sensation and autonomic dysfunction. Peripheral vascular disease (atherosclerosis of large and/or small leg vessels) causes ischaemia. Trauma (which may involve altered pressure-loading and be unnoticed by the patient) followed by infection complicates neuropathy and ischaemia to cause significant tissue damage, such as ulceration.

There are two main pathological pathways in diabetic feet:

- *Neuropathic feet* have good circulation (pulses are present) and are warm, dry, numb and usually painless. The two main complications are neuropathic ulcers (commonly on the soles) and neuropathic (Charcot) joints. Rapidly spreading infection can result in massive tissue destruction, the main indication for amputation in neuropathic feet.

Table 8.8. Order of priorities for treatment of diabetic dyslipidaemia[7]

Main treatment aim	First choice	Second choice	Third choice
LDL-C lowering	Statin	Anion-exchange resin or fibrate	
HDL-C raising	Behavioural: weight loss; increased exercise; smoking cessation	Difficult: nicotinic acid (with caution) *or* fibrate	
Triglyceride lowering	Optimal glycaemic control	Fibrate	Statin at high dose (especially if raised LDL)
Combined hyperlipidaemia	Optimal glycaemic control *plus* statin	Optimal glycaemic control *plus* statin *plus* fibrate*	Optimal glycaemic control *plus* statin *plus* nicotinic acid*

*The combination of a statin with nicotinic acid or, especially, a fibrate may increase the risk of myositis.

- *Neuro-ischaemic feet* are also numb, but cool, and the pulses are absent. In addition to the above neuropathic complications, pain at rest, ulcers at the edges, which result from trauma such as pressure damage, and gangrene may occur.

In both groups, the sequence of minor trauma, cutaneous ulceration and finally failure of the wound to heal can lead to amputation.

A UK population-based study in type 2 patients gave a prevalence of 1.4% for foot ulcers, but the prevalence of the risk factors that give rise to ulcers was 41.6%.[52] Up to 50% of foot ulcers and amputations could be prevented by patient education and effective intervention.[53] Once a limb has been amputated the prognosis for the contralateral limb is poor.[54] It was estimated that the total annual cost of treating diabetic foot problems in the UK in 1994 was £13 million.[55] Foot ulcers are more common in Caucasians than in Indo-Asians or Afro-Caribbeans, and are associated with adverse social circumstances (deprivation and isolation),[53] poor glycaemic control, the presence of other vascular risk factors (e.g., smoking) and increased duration of diabetes.

Targets

The targets are:
- Patient education to provide effective primary prevention, and prompt appropriate illness-seeking behaviour in the presence of suspected pathology;
- Identification of patients who have either a high risk (presence of neuropathy and/or peripheral vascular disease) of developing, or the presence of, lower-limb complications (e.g., foot ulcer, gangrene); and
- Optimal management of these identified patients to minimise morbidity, especially amputation.

Table 8.9. Relevant history in evaluation of diabetic foot problems

Patient's level of understanding of preventative foot care
Elicit sensory symptoms: pain, numbness, coldness, tingling
Previous history of foot ulcer(s)
Visual acuity; neuropathy is more prevalent in type 2 diabetics with retinopathy, which
    carries an increased risk of injury during self-care
Social circumstances

Who assesses?
The GP, practice nurse or podiatrist makes the assessment.

Evaluation
The evaluation should be systematic and form part of a structured foot-care pathway. The aim is to determine the level of risk to the diabetic foot and, thus, to indicate the appropriate management. The stages of the evaluation are to take a history (*Table 8.9*), carry out an examination (*Table 8.10*) and categorise the level of risk (*Table 8.11*).

Table 8.10. Examination of the diabetic foot

Inspect footwear for suitability and for evidence of excessive wear or pressure loading
Inspect distal lower limbs, looking for:
- Foot deformity, callus formation at pressure areas (increased risk of trauma)
- Distended foot veins (associated with autonomic neuropathy)
- Small muscle wasting (associated with somatic neuropathy)
- Oedema (associated with impaired circulation)
- Hair loss (associated with impaired circulation)
- Colour changes (pallor associated with ischaemia; erythema associated with cellulitis)
- Ulcerative lesions (neuropathic more likely on the sole; ischaemic more likely on the toe tips and/or dorsum)
- Other serious lesions, such as abscess, osteomyelitis or gangrene

Check for evidence of neuropathy:
- Decreased vibration sensation using a 128Hz tuning fork, or a biothesiometer (if available)
- Decreased skin pressure perception threshold using a 10g (5.07) monofilament, which is pushed perpendicularly against the skin on the sole of the foot until it buckles; inability to feel the filament applied in this way indicates a greater risk of developing a foot ulcer[56]
- Decreased ankle reflexes
- Dry and warm skin may indicate autonomic neuropathy

Check for evidence of impaired circulation:
- Reduced or absent pulses: in proximal disease femoral pulses are weak and more distal pulses are absent; in distal disease, which occurs more often in diabetics, femoral and popliteal pulses are normal, but foot pulses are absent
- Decreased skin temperature
- Foot whitens when held elevated for 30 seconds
- If available, Doppler can be used to quantify the extent of arterial obstruction by measuring blood pressure in the lower limb

Check for evidence of musculoskeletal abnormalities:
- Is the range of movement of ankle joint and foot normal?
- Analysis of gait and stance abnormalities may suggest trauma and/or tissue damage

The structured examination of a diabetic foot should aim to identify any evidence of:

- Neuropathy, circulatory impairment or abnormal pressure that puts the foot 'at risk';
- A serious diabetic foot problem, such as ulcer, infection (cellulitis, abscess and/or osteomyelitis) or gangrene.

Table 8.12 summarises a longer-established classification of diabetic foot lesions that is useful in secondary care, although it does not categorise risk.

Interventions

The level of risk to the diabetic foot, as categorised in *Table 8.11*, indicates the optimal management pathway. Prompt and decisive intervention, such as early referral, intravenous antibi-

Table 8.11. Summary of assessment and indicated management pathways for diabetic feet*

Level of risk	Assessment findings	Interventions
Low risk	Normal sensation *and good pulses;* no previous ulcer; no foot deformity; normal vision	No specific podiatrist input Trained patient undertakes own nail care Review in 12 months
Moderate risk	Loss of sensation *or* Absent pulses (or previous vascular surgery) *or* Significant visual impairment *or* Physical disability (e.g., cardiovascular accident, gross obesity)	Regular podiatry (at 4–12 week intervals) Interim review at 2-6 months
High risk	Previous ulcer caused by neuropathy and/or ischaemia *or* Absent pulses *and* neuropathy *or* Callus with risk factor (neuropathy, absent pulse, foot deformity) *or* Previous amputation	Refer to podiatrist with special interest in diabetes *or* Refer to local hospital-based specialist diabetes team
Active foot disease	Active foot ulceration *or* Painful neuropathy difficult to control	Contact local hospital-based specialist diabetes team for urgent appointment
Emergency foot problem	*Critical ischaemia,* as characterised by: rest or night pain *or* pale/mottled foot *or* dependent rubor *or* ischaemic ulceration *or* gangrene *Severe infection,* as characterised by: abscess *or* cellulitis	Emergency referral to hospital

*Adapted from the Tayside foot risk assessment protocol quoted in the Scottish Intercollegiate Guidelines Network.[57]

Table 8.12. Classification of diabetic foot lesions[58]

Grade	Description
0	High-risk foot; no ulcers
1	Superficial ulcer (skin deep), not clinically infected
2	Deeper ulcer, often with cellulitis; no abscess or bony involvement
3	Deep ulcer with abscess or bony involvement (osteomyelitis)
4	Localised gangrene (involving toe, forefoot or heel)
5	Gangrene of the entire foot

otics or angioplasty when indicated, reduces the risk of progression to a higher-grade lesion (as in *Table 8.12*) and, ultimately and regrettably, amputation. Patients with peripheral vascular disease probably have widespread atheroma and therefore are at a higher risk of having developing cardiovascular disease, which needs to be addressed in any management plan.

Suitable interventions carried out in the primary care setting may include:

- Advice by the GP, nurse or podiatrist (following the guidance set out in *Table 8.13*);
- Debridement. Patients with neuropathic ulcers require removal of any dead skin or callus. This should be carried out by a suitably qualified podiatrist only.
- Prescription:
  - Aspirin reduces cardiovascular mortality, and should be considered if there are no contraindications.
  - A broad-spectrum antibiotic should be prescribed for infections. The choice should be guided by culture, sensitivity results (where available) and response to treatment. A longer duration and higher dose of antibiotic is usually required because of the poorer tissue perfusion and delayed healing that occurs in diabetics.
  - If the neuropathic ulcer does not heal after debridement, good evidence now supports the topical use of growth factors (RGD peptide[60] and CT-102[61]) or of becaplermin[62] to quicken healing rates. However, these treatments are extremely expensive and should be undertaken only by specialists.
  - Neuropathic pain does not respond to conventional analgesia. Tricyclic antidepressants, the anticonvulsant carbamazepine, and topical capsaicin can be effective in reducing pain. Gabapentin is another anticonvulsant that increasingly is being used successfully by pain management experts (see the section below on neuropathy for a fuller discussion).
- Improved glycaemic control (see above).
- Improved management of other vascular risk factors (optimal blood pressure, smoking cessation, better lipid profile).

Referral to secondary care (according to the level of risk categorised in *Table 8.11*) may lead to the following interventions:

- Custom-built footwear or orthotic insoles should be used to reduce plantar callus thickness and the incidence of foot ulcer relapse in high-risk diabetic feet.
- Patients with tissue loss and arterial disease should be considered for arterial reconstruction or angioplasty by a vascular surgeon. These are more likely to succeed in proximal disease than in the more common distal disease.

Table 8.13. Diabetic patient guidelines for foot care[59]

Hygiene

Good hygiene is essential: twice-weekly bathing and gentle dryings are recommended; socks or stockings should be changed daily, the foot inspected carefully for infection and talc avoided

How to avoid problems

Do not wear constricting footwear

Do not walk bare foot, sit by an open fire or use hot water bottles

Do not wear garters; these can reduce blood supply to the feet

Do not treat your own corns or callosities; go to a state-registered podiatrist

Do not cut your toenails if you have difficulty in managing; cut nails straight across and not too short

Examine feet regularly for possible injuries, using a mirror to inspect the soles

Shoes should be inspected before and after putting them on; ensure no grit or other objects are in the shoe; avoid wear of lining, insoles and heels

Proper fitting and selection are essential when buying new shoes (measure feet when standing; uppers should be of soft leather; ensure enough room across the ball of the foot and around the toes to enable wiggling; there should be some sort of fastening mechanism; soles should be of rubber or microcellular type; avoid excessively high heels); high-quality cushioned-sole trainers reduce plantar pressure more than ordinary shoes, but not as much as custom-built shoes

Keep feet warm in winter: natural fibre cotton and/or wool hosiery is better than nylon

Seek advice from your podiatrist or doctor if you notice:
    any foot injuries
    any swelling or throbbing pain in any part of your feet
    any colour changes in any part of your feet
    any discharge of coloured fluid from your feet, especially from corns, calluses or
      beneath toenails
    undue numbness or prickling sensation in your feet

- Redistribution of weight using casts may be used to protect the vulnerable foot. In the case of Charcot's foot (a neuroarthropathic process with osteoporosis, fracture, acute inflammation and disorganised foot architecture), total contact casting and nonweight bearing are effective treatments.

Following discharge from hospital, the GP or practice nurse must monitor closely these patients and continue to undertake the above-stated primary care interventions.

Eyes

As with foot care, any programme for the screening and management of diabetic eye disease should be structured.

Rationale

Diabetes mellitus has long been associated with eye problems, including retinopathy, cataracts and glaucoma. Individually or collectively, these can give rise to visual loss. The St Vincent Declaration of 1989 set a target to reduce new blindness caused by diabetes by one-third or more.[51] For type 2 patients, glaucoma and cataracts are more important than retinopathy in causing visual loss, but retinopathy is already present in one-fifth of type 2 patients at diagnosis[20] and its prevalence is related directly to the duration of diabetes.

Among the risk factors associated with the development and progression of diabetic retinal disease in type 2 diabetics are: raised blood pressure,[28] increased duration of diabetes,[63] and the presence of microalbuminuria.[64]

Active management of micro-angiopathy affecting the retina has been possible since the development of photocoagulation. Cataract surgery and other surgical techniques that may benefit patients with diabetic eye disease are now available. Nevertheless, regular screening for diabetic disease should improve the prognosis, by detecting abnormalities earlier in their natural history. As discussed in the section on albuminuria, the presence of diabetic retinopathy is associated with diabetes-related renal disease.

Targets

The targets are:
- Early detection of treatable abnormalities in the lens and/or retina;
- Preservation of visual function.

Who assesses?

The two preferred methods of screening for retinopathy (meeting the clinical guidelines recommendation of a sensitivity of 80% or higher and a specificity of 95% or higher[65]) are:
- A suitably trained assessor (optician, GP with ophthalmological experience), ideally using mydriatic slit-lamp indirect ophthalmoscopy; or
- Mydriatic retinal photography (first choice), when undertaken by and when the images are evaluated by trained personnel.

If the practice does not have access to either a slit-lamp or a retinal photography service, suitably trained personnel only should screen retinas using direct ophthalmoscopy (an ophthalmoscope) with mydriasis, although the reported sensitivity and specificity are lower for this method than the recommended minimum above and it risks missing clinically significant macular oedema (CSMO).

The National Screening Committee recommended that diabetic retinopathy screening programmes should:
- Undertake an annual programme for all those with diabetes;
- Have an integral quality assurance framework;
- Be integrated with the other local programmes for diabetic care.

Retinopathy screening is an early high priority in the Diabetes NSF: the aim is to offer it to 80% of diabetics by March 2006, rising to 100% by the end of 2007 (see Chapter 1). The preferred screening methods are more likely to meet these criteria.

Evaluation

Visual acuity

To check visual acuity (not all retinopathy affects vision, especially if the macula is spared):

- Use a properly illuminated Snellen chart of correct size for 3 or 6 metres;
- Use a pinhole to correct refractory errors.

Fundoscopy

Before dilating pupils with 1% tropicamide, check:

- Depth of the anterior chambers (shining a torch from the side at a right angle should illuminate the whole of the iris) to exclude any increased risk of provoking acute angle closure;
- That the patient is aware that he or she should not drive for approximately 6 hours after the drops (although there is debate about the extent to which mydriasis can affect driving vision).

Allow at least 10 minutes for drops to work, after which check red reflex. Start with the ophthalmoscope 18 inches (50cm) in front of each eye, and adjust the focus to look for corneal scars, lens opacities and vitreous haemorrhage.

Examine the retina systematically:

- Start at the optic disc, looking for new vessels or cupping (evidence of glaucoma);
- Locate the macula and check the surrounding area for haemorrhages and exudates (especially hard exudates in a circular pattern);
- Follow the major veins from the optic disc out to the periphery looking for venous irregularities (e.g., beading) and new vessels;
- Inspect elsewhere in the retina for haemorrhages (micro-, intraretinal or larger), exudates ('soft' or 'hard'), fibrous tissue or detachment.

The findings that determine the classification of diabetic retinopathy are outlined in *Figure 8.1.*

Intervention

The management of diabetic retinopathy follows the pathways outlined in *Table 8.14*. Suitable interventions in primary care are:

- *Modification of risk factors* (tighter glycaemic and blood pressure control; see the sections above for further details). It is advisable to stabilise sight-threatening retinal disease first, as rapid improvement in glycaemic control can result in the short-term worsening of diabetic retinal disease. However, tight blood glucose control has been shown to reduce the progression of diabetic retinopathy (needing requiring retinal photocoagulation) and the deterioration of visual acuity in type 2 diabetics.[9] Aspirin use, in the absence of contraindications, should be considered (see Chapter 9).
- *Appropriate referral to secondary care*, depending upon the degree of retinopathy found or whether cataracts interfere with vision.
- *Rehabilitation* may involve community support, low vision aids and training in their use for patients with visual impairment.

Secondary-care interventions may include the following:

- *Laser photocoagulation* for high-risk retinopathy (moderately proliferative or worse) and CSMO (focal or modified grid laser);
- *Vitrectomy* may be considered in type 2 diabetics who have a vitreous haemorrhage too severe to allow laser photocoagulation;
- *Cataract extraction*, the outcome of which is closely linked to age and severity of retinopathy present before surgery.

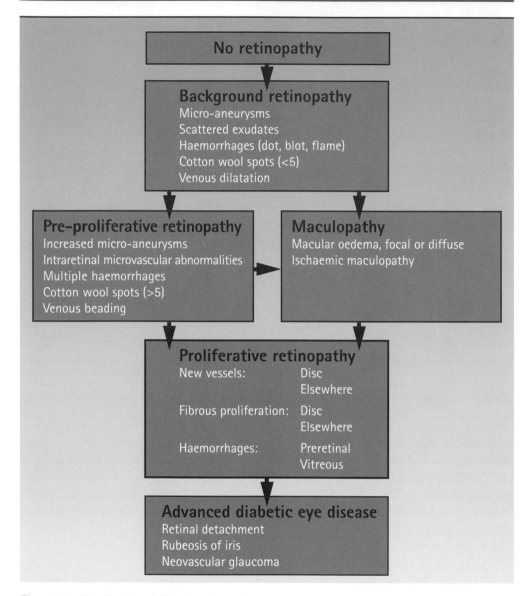

Figure 8.1. Classification of diabetic retinopathy.

Albuminuria

Rationale

Raised urine albumin levels may be associated with nephropathy in patients with diabetes. If retinopathy is also present, diabetes-related renal disease is the likely cause of the albuminuria. If retinopathy is absent, other causes of renal disease should be considered.[67] Persistent macroalbuminuria (albumin excretion greater than 300mg/day) in the absence of infection marks the onset of diabetic nephropathy, and is also associated with increased mortality, particularly from vascular causes.[68] The natural history of overt diabetic nephropathy is to progress to end-stage renal failure, of which the prevalence is increasing. Indo-Asian and Afro-Caribbean type 2 diabetics appear to be at a greater risk of developing diabetic nephropathy than do Caucasian type 2 diabetics.

Table 8.14. Management pathways following eye assessment[66]

Care pathway	Visual acuity	Lens	Retina*	Other factors
Routine review (1 year)	Unchanged	Clear or Minimal opacities	No changes or Minimal/low risk background	
Early review (3–6 months)			New or worsening lesions or Exudates >1 dd from fovea	Renal disease or Rapid improvement of blood glucose
Routine referral to ophthalmologist		Cataracts interfering with vision	View is obscured (but beware of possibility of significant retinopathy)	
Rapid referral (within 4 weeks) to ophthalmologist	Unexplained drop		Hard exudates <1 dd from fovea or Macular oedema or Unexplained findings or Pre-proliferative retinopathy or More advanced (severe) retinopathy	
Urgent referral (within 1 week) to ophthalmologist			New vessels	Pre-retinal and/or vitreous haemorrhage Rubeosis iridis
Emergency referral (same day) to ophthalmologist	Sudden loss		Retinal detachment	

*dd, disc diameter.

Target

To identify and manage patients at increased risk of premature vascular disease and of diabetic nephropathy, and to reduce their risk of progressing to end-stage renal failure.

Microalbuminuria

The presence of lesser amounts of urinary albumin (<300mg/day), termed microalbuminuria, indicates early renal damage. This is now recognised as a risk factor for cardiovascular morbidity and mortality in type 2 diabetics.[69] The 'gold standard' for the diagnosis of microalbuminuria is the albumin excretion rate (AER) in a timed urine sample, but this is not a practical screening procedure in the community. Collecting an early morning urine sample to be sent to a chemical pathology laboratory to measure the albumin:creatinine ratio (ACR) is both more practical and the preferred method recommended by the ARA.[70]

ACR levels equal to or greater than 2.5mg/mmol in males or 3.5mg/mmol in females indicate likely microalbuminuria. The test needs to be repeated for confirmation, as microalbuminuria can be transient. The author recently completed a study in which he found that the prevalence of microalbuminuria in diabetics in an ethnically mixed UK community to be about 19.3% (with a 95% confidence interval of 17.2–21.4%). The characteristics independently associated with a higher prevalence of microalbuminuria were current insulin use, current smoking, older age, higher systolic blood pressure and poorer metabolic control, but there was no significant association with either increasing duration or gender. Unfortunately, the sample size was not large enough to determine whether there was an association between microalbuminuria and Indo-Asian ethnicity.[71]

The implementation of screening for microalbuminuria requires evidence that intervention will benefit those who screen positive (the principles of screening are discussed in Chapter 4). There is abundant and solid evidence that, in normotensive type 1 diabetes patients with microalbuminuria, drugs that inhibit the renin–angiotensin–aldosterone system (ACE inhibitors and angiotensin-receptor blockers) delay the progression of renal nephropathy, independently of their lowering blood pressure. Recent reports suggest that angiotensin-receptor blockers are reno-protective in type 2 diabetics with either hypertension and microalbuminuria[72] or more overt nephropathy.[73,74] Regrettably, these trials did not test the more established and less expensive ACE inhibitors. Further evidence is required to determine which type 2 diabetics (level of blood pressure, degree of nephropathy, ethnic group) would benefit from drugs that inhibit the renin–angiotensin–aldosterone system (ACE inhibitors or angiotensin-receptor blockers or both).

Who assesses?
The GP or practice nurse makes the assessment.

Evaluation
Macroalbuminuria screening should be undertaken, using a suitable test strip on a urine sample. The ADA recommends microalbuminuria screening in all type 2 diabetics, sending off an early morning sample to measure ACR.[70] The latest NICE guidelines recommend either of the above methods.[23] If albuminuria is found, an infection needs to be excluded. After an infection has been treated, the screening needs to be repeated.

Intervention
If albuminuria is found, the following may delay or prevent deterioration in renal function:
• Tight blood pressure control, with increasing evidence to support the preferred use of drugs that inhibit the renin–angiotensin–aldosterone system (ACE inhibitors and ARAs);
• Optimal glycaemic control;
• Cessation of smoking;
• Correction of abnormal lipid profile;
Referral to an appropriate specialist is indicated either for further investigations or for management when diabetic nephropathy has progressed.

Serum creatinine
Rationale
A raised serum creatinine indicates renal impairment, most often caused by diabetes. It requires prompt and effective interventions (discussed below) to prevent end-stage renal failure.

Colour Plates

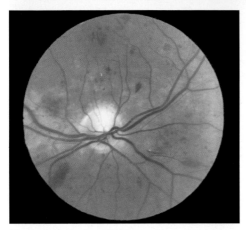

Plate 1. Background retinopathy.

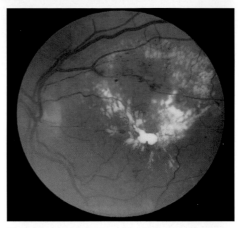

Plate 2. Maculopathy with circinate exudates.

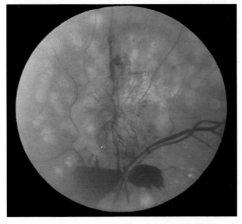

Plate 3. Proliferative retinopathy with disc new vessels and subhyloid haemorrhage.

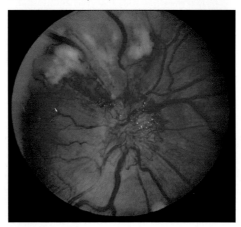

Plate 4. Proliferative retinopathy with disc new vessels.

Plate 5. Pre-proliferative retinopathy.

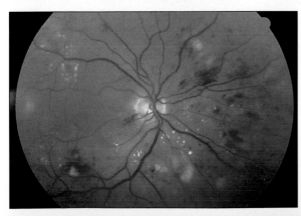

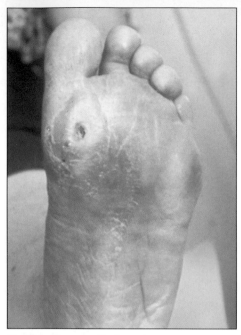

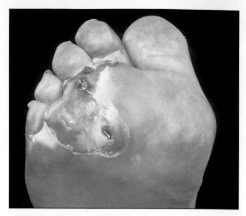

Plate 7. Neuropathic foot ulcer.

Plate 6. Neuropathic foot ulcer.

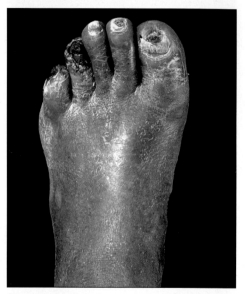

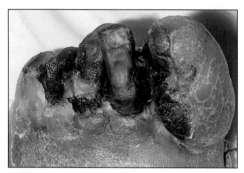

Plate 8. Gangrene with adjacent cellulites.

Plate 9. Ischaemic foot with digital gangrene.

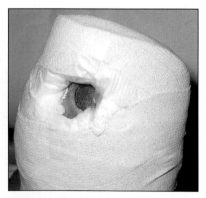

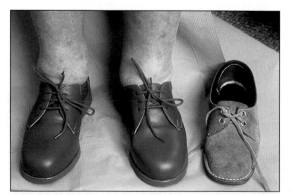

Plate 10. Scotchcast boot showing neuropathic ulcer under window.

Plate 11. Specialist diabetic footwear.

Target
Serum creatinine greater than 120nmol/l indicates renal impairment.

Who assesses?
The GP or practice nurse makes the assessment.

Evaluation
A blood test for serum creatinine (often referred to as 'U & Es') can be ordered from the local chemical pathology laboratory. Reference values may vary between different laboratories, but creatinine levels in ranges between 120 and 300nmol/l, 300 and 700nmol/l and above 700nmol/l indicate, respectively, mild, moderate and severe renal impairment. Checking the serum potassium at the same time can be useful. Hyperkalaemia (serum potassium above the upper reference limit – usually 5.5mEq/l) can result from ACE inhibitors and may occur in renal impairment. Hypokalaemia (serum potassium below the lower reference limit, usually 3.5mEq/l) can result from long-term thiazide treatment without potassium-sparing medication or supplement.

Intervention
Any nondiabetic causes of renal impairment should be identified and managed appropriately. To prevent further deterioration, tight glycaemic and blood pressure control are critical. Patients should be advised about their diet and to stop smoking. Referral to either the diabetic clinic or to a nephrologist should be considered if there is evidence of renal impairment.

Any cause of abnormal serum potassium should also be identified and managed appropriately. If iatrogenic, treatment should be corrected to restore normokalaemia.

Neuropathy
Rationale
Diabetic neuropathy is a common complication. It can cause considerable morbidity and may contribute to premature mortality. A possible hypothesis for the biochemical basis of diabetic neuropathy is discussed in Chapter 3. Neuropathies result from microangiopathy of the vasa nervorum. The development of diabetic neuropathy starts with *intraneural biochemical abnormalities*, which lead to *decreased nerve conduction velocity*, then to *clinical neuropathy* and end with *end-stage complications* caused by major irreversible derangements of the nerve structure and function. Many cases do not progress through all of the stages, and only the latter two stages are clinically apparent. A classification and the clinical features of diabetic neuropathy are given in *Table 8.15*.

Target(s)
The targets are:
- Prevent or delay the onset of further neuropathy;
- Alleviate symptoms (e.g., pain).

Who assesses?
The GP or practice nurse makes the assessment.

Evaluation
Before attributing the neuropathy found to diabetes, nondiabetic causes of neuropathy should be considered, including uraemia, deficiencies (B12), alcohol, neoplasia, paraproteinaemia,

Table 8.15. Classification and features of diabetic neuropathies[75]

Type of neuropathy	Features include
Peripheral sensorimotor	(Acute or chronic) symmetrical; mainly sensory Pain is sharp, stabbing or burning Paraesthesia of soles or hyperaesthesia Often has a stocking-glove distribution
Autonomic: postural hypotension gustatory sweating gastroparesis change in bowel frequency erectile dysfunction (see below)	Dizziness Abnormal facial sweating while eating Nausea and vomiting Diarrhoea (often nocturnal) or constipation
Mononeuropathy: external nerve pressure	Median carpal tunnel syndrome Cranial nerves (III, IV, VI, VII) Radial, ulnar and peroneal nerve palsies associated with pain
Proximal motor	Severe pain, associated with poor control Paraesthesiae in the proximal lower limbs Muscle wasting

Guillain–Barré syndrome and drugs such as nitrofurantoin. Nausea, vomiting and diarrhoea can be caused by infection.

The diagnosis of diabetic neuropathy is mainly clinical, so specialised investigations are usually unnecessary. Based upon the features listed in *Table 8.15*, a brief screening history should elicit the presence of both suspicious symptoms, such as pain, weakness, sensory dysfunction, sweating or gastrointestinal dysfunction (nausea, vomiting and/or diarrhoea), and of any features that suggest a nondiabetic cause. The examination is influenced by the history. Ankle jerks are usually decreased or absent in peripheral sensorimotor diabetic neuropathy (polyneuropathy), which is usually present if autonomic neuropathy occurs. A decreased heart rate in response to the Valsalva manoeuvre and/or an unchanged heart rate variation during deep breathing is evidence of autonomic neuropathy.

Intervention

The optimal management of diabetic neuropathy depends to some extent upon its type and presentation. Care should be taken to monitor any side effects of any medication used. Management options for different neuropathies include the following:

* In all cases, *good glycaemic control* may improve or delay worsening of neuropathy. Any underlying causes should be treated where possible.
* *Analgesia.* Neuropathic pain does not respond to conventional analgesia. The first-line drugs are the tricyclic antidepressants (e.g., amitriptyline, imipramine and desipramine). The anticonvulsants carbamazepine and phenytoin are second-line drugs, and topical capsaicin can be effec-

tive. Gabapentin is another anticonvulsant that is being used increasingly, with success, by pain-management experts. Proximal motor neuropathic pain may be relieved by amitriptyline.

- *Other drug therapies.* Postural hypotension may respond to elevation of the head of the bed or to fludrocortisone (beware of hypertension and/or oedema). Anticholinergics, such as propantheline, may relieve gustatory sweating. Metoclopramide, domperidone and cis-apride have been used to treat gastroparesis.
- *Psychological support* is important, especially when the neuropathy is disabling.
- *Rehabilitation and education* may be helpful, particularly when there is motor impairment.
- Mononeuropathies (i.e., cranial nerve) often *improve spontaneously* within weeks to months.
- If the primary care team has no success and the patient is still troubled, *referral* to either a diabetologist or a pain clinic is indicated.
- Some mononeuropathies caused by external compression (e.g., carpal tunnel) can be treated by *surgical decompression* with a good prognosis.
- Appropriate *treatment of nondiabetic causes* of neuropathy.

Erectile dysfunction

Rationale

Sexual dysfunction is an important and common problem in diabetic men, but other causes need to be considered and treated, if appropriate.[76]

Target

To restore or compensate for sexual dysfunction in accordance with the patient's wishes.

Who assesses?

The GP or practice nurse makes the assessment.

Evaluation

History

The history should be elicited tactfully, aiming to define the dysfunction and to identify any possible contributory factors. If there is a partner, his or her presence is helpful. Relevant areas to question are:

- *Nature of the dysfunction.* Is it lack of tumescence or early collapse of erection or both? How long has it been going on, and did it start suddenly or gradually? Do spontaneous or early morning erections ever occur? Is libido normal and sexual stimulation present? Is there a problem with orgasm and ejaculation, and what is considered normal? Details of the current relationship, the partner's attitude and the couple's expectations. What remedies have been tried already?
- Relevant *current medical history* (apart from diabetes), looking for endocrine abnormalities (hair loss, gynaecomastia, weight gain and change in heat tolerance), vascular disease (exercise-related chest or leg pain, if not already sought) and neurological disorder (problems with sensation, co-ordination and motor function).
- Relevant *past medical history*, particularly about pelvic surgery, radiotherapy or trauma, and psychiatric or psychological problems.
- *Medication.* Many drugs can cause erectile dysfunction, including thiazide diuretics, beta-blockers, antidepressants, tranquillisers, anxiolytics and H2 antagonists.

- *Lifestyle.* As well as smoking and alcohol, ask about recent major life changes and the use of recreational or bodybuilding drugs.

Information from the above should provide strong clues as to the origin of the dysfunction. Sudden onset, the presence of some erections, ejaculatory problems and major life events and/or psychological problems suggest a psychogenic cause, whereas gradual onset, no tumescence, the presence of risk factors, a past history of pelvic disease or treatment, certain medication or illicit drug use, smoking and heavy alcohol consumption suggest an organic cause.

Examination

For most patients, examination can be limited to the genitalia, looking for abnormalities in testicular size, fibrosis in the penile shaft and the retractability of the foreskin if present. Further examination, such as looking for the presence of secondary sexual characteristics (e.g., breasts, beard growth) may be indicated by the history.

Investigations

Further investigations are indicated by the findings of the history and examination. A free serum testosterone is the preferred screening investigation for suspected hypogonadism. Extensive endocrine investigations are usually unnecessary.

Intervention

Patients may not always be enthusiastic about medical intervention. Treatable underlying causes, such as medication, should be corrected, glycaemic control needs to be optimised and smoking should be discouraged. Counselling for psychological difficulties and clear unbiased information about treatment options, respecting patients' wishes, can be offered in general practice.

Referral should be considered to:

- *Urologist* if the patient has never had an erection and/or if there is a severe vascular problem and/or if the patient opts for an intervention beyond the practitioner's competence.
- *Psychosexual therapy* if the psychogenic component is significant. Often the waiting list for such therapy is very long and other appropriate therapeutic interventions should be considered in the meantime.
- *Endocrinologist* if a hormone abnormality is found, although treatment may not restore potency.

Sildenafil (Viagra) was the first available oral drug for the treatment of erectile dysfunction, with a reported improvement in 50–88% of patients. It selectively inhibits phosphodiesterase 5, an enzyme that breaks down cyclic guanosine monophosphate (GMP), an intracellular second messenger that produces smooth muscle relaxation and maintains penile blood flow. Sildenafil has no effect on the libido and does not produce an erection in the absence of sexual stimulation. Its contraindications are severe hepatic impairment, hypotension (blood pressure <90/50mmHg), recent stroke or myocardial infarction, hereditary degenerative retinal disorders and concurrent treatment with nitrates, nitric oxide donors and ritonavir [human immunodeficiency virus (HIV) protease inhibitor]. It should be prescribed with caution in penile deformity, conditions predisposing to priapism and if concurrent treatment with cimetidine, erythromycin, ketoconazole, itraconazole and other HIV protease inhibitors. Its side effects are mild and include headache, flushing, dyspepsia through relaxation of the oesophageal sphincter, and transient visual disturbances, which consist of a bluish tinge to white colours and last less than 20 minutes. Having provoked a major debate about rationing, sildenafil has been available from 1 July 1999 on NHS prescription to diabetic men with erectile dysfunction. It is formulated in doses of 25mg, 50mg and 100mg, marketed in packs of one, four, eight or 12 tablets, and is currently the cheapest treatment option. The maximum quantity that can be prescribed on the NHS is one tablet per week. The initial recommended dose is 50mg, reduced to 25mg in the elderly and in those with moderate hepatic impairment or severe renal failure. The dose may be increased to 100mg if necessary and if tolerated. Sildenafil should be taken 1 hour before sexual activity and not repeated within 24 hours. It is likely that other oral drugs for erectile dysfunction will become available soon.

Apomorphine (Uprima) is a dopamine agonist that activates specific neural events in the paraventricular nucleus of the hypothalamus. Oxytocinergic pathways then relax smooth muscle in the corpus cavernosum, which leads to erection within 20 minutes of use. Apomorphine can be prescribed on the NHS under the same conditions as sildenafil. The dose is one sublingual tablet of 2 or 3mg, not to be repeated within 8 hours.

Other currently licensed treatments should be considered if either sildenafil or apomorphine is contraindicated, unsuitable or ineffective. These include intracavernosal prostaglandin (alprostadil) injections, transurethral alprostadil (Muse), vacuum devices and penile prostheses. Referral to a suitable specialist clinic is usually warranted for these treatments.

Injection sites
Rationale
Injecting insulin into abnormal subcutaneous tissue may affect the proportion that reaches the circulation and its timing, and thus affect glycaemic control and make the evaluation of and response to plasma glucose levels more problematic. In addition, the presence of infection at injection sites can affect health.

Target
To ensure adequate injection technique and site selection.

Who assesses?
The practice nurse or GP makes the assessment.

Evaluation
For evaluation, the patient's injection technique is observed, and injection sites are inspected for atrophy or infection.

Intervention
If the injection technique is faulty, it must be corrected (details on insulin injections are given in Chapter 7). Any infected sites should be treated with antibiotics or referred to the diabetic clinic. An earlier review may be necessary.

Administration

Follow-up
Rationale
A regular review improves the quality and outcomes of diabetic care.

Targets
The targets are:

- 12 months for the next full periodic review;
- 2 to 6 months for the next interim check, depending upon the outcomes of the individual components of the review.

Who assesses?
Those who carried out the review make the assessment.

Evaluation
The evaluation depends upon the findings and interventions agreed for the individual components of the review.

Intervention
After agreeing with the patient, the interval for follow-up is documented in the medical records and the practice member responsible for organising the diabetic clinic recall informed.

Medication review
Rationale
From a clinical point of view, this is an ideal opportunity to ensure that the patient is being prescribed an optimal combination and quantity of both diabetic and nondiabetic medication (where applicable) and to ascertain compliance. From an administrative point of view, the correct and uninterrupted provision of repeat prescriptions can be ensured. Finally, this allows patients an opportunity to raise any queries or concerns that they may have about their medication, and the prescriber to check the patients' knowledge and understanding of treatment.

Target
The patient's repeat-prescriptions record accurately reflects the medication that should be taken and that the patient has sufficient supplies.

Who assesses?
The GP makes the assessment.

Evaluation
The evaluation involves a review of the prescription record (easy if prescriptions are issued by computer) and a check with patients of the details and dose of medication prescribed.

Intervention
After correcting the record, set a medication review date in the diary for a suitable interval, according to the practice's prescription protocol.

Data entry
Rationale
Accurate and complete information in the medical records facilitates patient care, enables audit and is a medico-legal requirement.

Target
The target is to ensure the data in the patient record are accurate, complete and accessible.

Who assesses?
The professional who carries out the periodic review makes the assessment.

Evaluation
Evaluation is mainly self-monitoring, but some practices may have in place some form of quality control, whereby medical records are scrutinised regularly for the quality of the entries.

Interventions
It may be advantageous to record all the relevant data on a template for either electronic or manual records systems. In addition to the information collected from carrying out the above components, it is necessary to record the date, who carried out the review and where it was done (clinic, home visit).

Key Points in this Chapter

- Regular review facilitates collaboration between each diabetic and the involved health care professional(s), and aims to optimise glycaemic control, modify risk factors for vascular disease and identify and minimise the effect of diabetic complications.

- A full periodic review should be undertaken once annually. Less comprehensive interim reviews should be undertaken at 2–6 month intervals.

- The components of the full review are divided into four sections: glycaemic control, risk factors/lifestyle, diabetic complications and administration.

REFERENCES

1 NICE Guideline Development Group and Recommendations Panel. *Inherited Clinical Guideline H. Management of type 2 diabetes: Management of blood pressure and blood lipids*. London: NHS National Institute for Clinical Excellence, 2002. Online: http://www.nice.org.uk

2 Law MR, Wald NJ. Risk factor thresholds: their existence under scrutiny. *BMJ* 2002; **324**: 1370–1376.

3 NICE Guideline Development Group and Recommendations Panel. *Inherited Clinical Guideline G. Management of type 2 diabetes: Management of blood glucose*. London: NHS National Institute for Clinical Excellence, 2002. Online: http://www.nice.org.uk

4 Rohlfing CL, Wiedmeyer HM, Little RR *et al*. Defining the relationship between plasma glucose and HbA1c analysis of glucose profiles and HbA1c in the Diabetes Control and Complications Trial. *Diabetes Care* 2002; 25; 275–278.

5 UK Prospective Diabetes Study Group. Intensive blood-glucose control with sulphonylureas or insulin compared with conventional treatment and risk of complications in patients with type 2 diabetes (UKPDS 33). *Lancet* 1998; **352**: 837–853.

6 European Diabetes Policy Group. A desktop guide to type 2 diabetes mellitus. *Diabet Med* 1999; **16**: 716–730.

7 American Diabetes Association: Position Statement. Standards of medical care for patients with diabetes mellitus. *Diabetes Care* 2003; **26**(Suppl. 1): S33–S50.

8 Winocour PH. Effective diabetes care: a need for realistic targets. *BMJ* 2002; **324**: 1577–1580.

9 Stratton IM, Adler AI, Neil HAW, *et al*. Association of glycaemia with macrovascular and microvascular complications of type 2 diabetes (UKPDS 35): prospective observational study. *BMJ* 2000; **321**: 405–412.

10 Toeller, M. Diet and diabetes. *Diabet Med* 1993: **9**(2): 15–18.

11 Leicestershire Health. *Dietary Recommendations for Adults with Diabetes in Leicestershire*. Leicester: Leicestershire Health Authority, 1997.

12 Peirce NS. Diabetes and exercise. *Br J Sports Med* 1999; **33**: 161–173.

13 Buckley J, Holmes J, Mapp G. *Exercise on Prescription: Cardiovascular Activity for Health*. Oxford: Butterworth–Heinemann, 1999.

14 American Diabetes Association. Clinical Practice Recommendations 2000: Diabetes mellitus and exercise. *Diabetes Care* 2003; **26** (Suppl. 1): S73–S77.

15 Ha T, Lean MEJ. Diet and lifestyle modification in the management of non-insulin-dependent diabetes mellitus. In: Pickup JC, Williams G, Eds. *Textbook of Diabetes*, 2nd Edn. Oxford: Blackwell Scientific, 1997: 37.14–37.15.

16 Tuomilehto J, Lindstorm J, Eriksson JG, *et al.* for the Finnish Diabetes Prevention Study Group. Prevention of type 2 diabetes mellitus by changes in lifestyle among subjects with impaired glucose tolerance. *N Engl J Med* 2001; **333**: 1343–1350.

17 American Diabetes Association. Diabetes and exercise: the risk–benefit profile. In: Devlin JT, Ruderman N, Eds. *The Health Professional's Guide to Diabetes and Exercise*. Alexandria: American Diabetes Association, 1995: 3–4.

18 Beers MH, Berkow R, Eds. *The Merck Manual of Diagnosis and Therapy*, 17th Edn. Whitehouse Station: Merck Research Laboratories, 1999.

19 Turner RC, Millns H, Neil HAW, *et al.* for the United Kingdom Prospective Diabetes Study Group. Risk factors for coronary artery disease in non-insulin-dependent diabetes mellitus: United Kingdom prospective diabetes study (UKPDS:23). *BMJ* 1998; **316**: 823–828.

20 Macleod CA, Munro J, Brameld K. *Health Gain Investment Programme Technical Review Document: Diabetes*. Sheffield: Trent Regional Health Authority, July 1994.

21 Prochaska JO, DiClemente CC. Stages of change in the modification of problem behaviors. *Prog Behav Modif.* 1992; **28**: 183–218.

22 Lancaster T, Stead L, Silagy C, *et al.* for the Cochrane Tobacco Addiction Review Group. Regular review: Effectiveness of interventions to help people stop smoking: findings from Cochrane. *BMJ* 2000; **321**: 355–358.

23 NICE Appraisal Committee. *Technology Appraisal Guidance No. 39: Guidance on the use of nicotine replacement therapy (NRT) and bupropion for smoking cessation*. London: NHS National Institute for Clinical Excellence, 2002. Online: http://www.nice.org.uk

24 The University of York and NHS Centre for Reviews and Dissemination. Smoking cessation: What the health service can do. *Effectiveness Matters* 1998; **3**.

25 Silagy C, Mant D, Fowler G, *et al.* Nicotine replacement therapy for smoking cessation. In: *Cochrane Library*. Oxford: Update Software, 1998; issue 2.

26 Joint Formulary Committee. *British National Formulary 44*. London: British Medical Association and Royal Pharmaceutical Society of Great Britain, 2002.

27 Hutchinson A, McIntosh A, Griffiths CJ, *et al. Clinical Guidelines and Evidence Review for Type 2 Diabetes. Blood pressure management*. Sheffield: ScHARR, University of Sheffield, 2002. Online: http://shef.ac.uk/guidelines

28 UK Prospective Diabetes Study Group. Tight blood pressure control and risk of macro vascular and micro vascular complications in type 2 diabetes: UKPDS 38. *BMJ* 1998; **317**: 703–712.

29 American Diabetes Association: Position Statement. Treatment of hypertension in adults with diabetes. *Diabetes Care* 2003; **26** (Suppl. 1): S80–S82.

30 O'Brien E, Beevers G, Lip GYH. ABC of hypertension. Blood pressure measurement. Part IV. Automated sphygmomanometry: self blood pressure measurement. *BMJ* 2001; **322**: 1167–1170.

31 UK Prospective Diabetes Study Group. Efficacy of atenolol and captopril in reducing risk of macro vascular and micro vascular complications in type 2 diabetes: UKPDS 39. *BMJ* 1998; **317**: 713–720.

32 ALLHAT Collaborative Research Group. Major outcomes in high-risk hypertensive patients randomized to angiotensin-converting enzyme inhibitor or calcium channel blocker vs diuretic: The Antihypertensive and Lipid-Lowering Treatment to Prevent Heart Attack Trial. *JAMA* 2002; **288**: 2981–2997.

33 The Heart Outcomes Prevention Evaluation Study Investigators. Effects of an angiotensin-converting-enzyme inhibitor, ramipril, on death from cardiovascular causes, myocardial infarction, and stroke in high-risk patients. *N Engl J Med* 2000; **342**: 145–153.

34 Dählof B, Devereux RB, Kjeldsen SE, *et al.* for the LIFE study group. Cardiovascular morbidity and mortality in the Losartan Intervention For Endpoint reduction in hypertension study (LIFE): a randomised trial against atenolol. *Lancet* 2002; **359**: 995–1003.

35 Mogensen CE, Neldam S, Tikkansen I, *et al.* for the CALM study group. Randomised control trial of dual blockade of the rennin–angiotensin system in patients with hypertension, microalbuminuria, and non-insulin dependent diabetes: the candesartan and lisinopril microalbuminuria (CALM) study. *BMJ* 2000; **321**: 1440–1444.

36 Estacio RO, Jeffers BW, Hiatt WR, *et al.* The effect of nisoldipine as compared with enalapril on cardiovascular events in patients with non-insulin-dependent diabetes and hypertension. *N Engl J Med* 1998; **338**: 645–652.

37 Ramsay LE, Williams B, Johnston GD, *et al.* British Hypertension Society guidelines for hypertension management 1999: summary. *BMJ* 1999; **319**: 630–635.

38 NICE Appraisal Committee. *Technology Appraisal Guidance No. 22: Guidance on the use of orlistat for the treatment of obesity in adults*. London: NHS National Institute for Clinical Excellence, 2001. Online: www.nice.org.uk

39 NICE Appraisal Committee. *Technology Appraisal Guidance No. 31: Guidance on the use of sibutramine for the treatment of obesity in adults*. London: NHS National Institute for Clinical Excellence, 2001. Online: www.nice.org.uk

40 McIntosh A, Hutchinson A, Feder G, *et al. Clinical Guidelines and Evidence Review for Type 2 Diabetes. Lipids management*. Sheffield: ScHARR, University of Sheffield, 2002. Online: http://shef.ac.uk/guidelines

41 Jones DB, Gill GV. Non-insulin dependent diabetes mellitus: an overview. In: Pickup JC, Williams G, Eds. *Textbook of Diabetes*, 2nd Edn. Oxford: Blackwell Scientific, 1997: 17.9.

42 Betteridge DJ. Lipid disorders in diabetes mellitus. In: Pickup JC, Williams G, Eds. *Textbook of Diabetes*, 2nd Edn. Oxford: Blackwell Scientific, 1997: Ch 55.

43 Collins R, Armitage J, Parish S, *et al.* for the Heart Protection Study Collaborative Group. MRC/BHF Heart Protection Study of cholesterol lowering with simvastatin in 20,536 high-risk individuals: a randomised placebo-controlled trial. *Lancet* 2002; **360**: 7–22.

44 British Cardiac Society, British Hyperlipidaemia Association, British Hypertension Society, and endorsed by the British Diabetic Association. Joint British recommendations on prevention of coronary heart disease in clinical practice. *Heart* 1998; **80** (Suppl. 2): S1–S29.

45 Expert Panel on Detection, Evaluation and Treatment of High Blood Cholesterol in Adults. Executive

summary of the Third Report of the National Cholesterol Education Program (NCEP) of high blood cholesterol in adults (Adult Treatment Panel III). *JAMA* 2001; **285**: 2486–2497.

46 Goldberg RB, Mellies MJ, Sacks FM, *et al.* Cardiovascular events and their reduction with pravastatin in diabetic and glucose-intolerant myocardial infarction survivors with average cholesterol levels: subgroup analyses in the cholesterol and recurrent events (CARE) trial. The Care Investigators. *Circulation* 1998; **98**: 2513–9.

47 Long-Term Intervention with Pravastatin in Ischaemic Disease (LIPID) Study Group. Prevention of cardiovascular events and death with pravastatin in patients with coronary heart disease and a broad range of initial cholesterol levels. *N Engl J Med* 1998; **339**: 1349–57

48 WOSCOPS. Influence of pravastatin and plasma lipids on clinical events in the West of Scotland Coronary Prevention Study (WOSCOPS). *Circulation* 1998; **97**: 1440–5

49 Scandinavian Simvastatin Survival Study. Randomised trial of cholesterol lowering in 4444 patients with coronary heart disease: the Scandinavian Simvastatin Survival Study (4S). *Lancet* 1994; **344**: 1383–9

50 Duncan C (Ed.) *Monthly Index of Medical Specialities.* London: Haymarket Medical Publishing, 2002.

51 Krans HMJ, Porta M, Keen H, *et al.* (Eds). *Diabetes Care and Research in Europe. The St Vincent Declaration Action Programme Implementation Document,* 2nd Edn. Copenhagen: World Health Organisation, Regional Office for Europe, 1995.

52 Kumar S, Ashe HA, Parnell LN, *et al.* The prevalence of foot ulceration and its correlates in Type 2 diabetic patients. *Diabet Med* 1994; **11**: 480–484.

53 Boulton AJM. The diabetic foot. *Medicine* 1997; **25**: 39–42.

54 Ebskov B, Josephsen P. Incidence of reamputation and death after gangrene of the lower extremity. *Prosthet Orthot Int* 1980; **4**: 77–80.

55 Williams DRR. The size of the problem; epidemiological and economic aspects of foot problems in diabetes. In: Boulton AJM, Conner H, Cavanagh PR, Eds. *The Foot in Diabetes*, 2nd Edn. Chichester: John Wiley and Sons, 1994: 15–24.

56 Hutchinson A, McIntosh A, Feder G, *et al. Clinical Guidelines for Type 2 Diabetes: Prevention and management of foot problems.* London: Royal College of General Practitioners, 2000.

57 Scottish Intercollegiate Guidelines Network. *Management of Diabetes: A National Clinical Guideline (Number 55).* Edinburgh: SIGN Executive, Royal College of Physicians, 2001. Online: www.sign.ac.uk

58 Wagner FW. Algorithms of diabetic foot care. In: Levin ME, O'Neil LW, Eds. *The Diabetic Foot*, 2nd Edn. St Louis: Mosby-Yearbook, 1983: 291–302.

59 Leicestershire Health. *The Leicestershire Handbook for Diabetes,* Leicester: Leicestershire Health Authority, 1996.

60 Steed DL, Ricotta JJ, Prendergast JJ, *et al.* Promotion and acceleration of diabetic ulcer healing by arginine–glycine–aspartic acid (RGD) peptide matrix. RGD Study Group. *Diabetes Care* 1995; **18**: 39–46.

61 Holloway G, Steed D, DeMarco M, *et al.* A randomised controlled dose response trial of activated platelet

supermatant, topical CT-102 in chronic, non-healing diabetic wounds. *Wound* 1993; **5**: 198–206.

62 Wierman TJ, Smiell JM, Su Y. Efficacy and safety of a topical gel formulation of recombinant human platelet-derived growth factor-BB (becaplermin) in patients with chronic neuropathic diabetic ulcers. A phase III randomized placebo-controlled double-blind study. *Diabetes Care* 1998; **21**: 822–827.

63 Klein R, Klein BE, Moss SE, *et al.* The Wisconsin epidemiologic study of diabetic retinopathy III. Prevalence and risk of diabetic retinopathy when age at diagnosis is 30 or more years. *Arch Ophthalmol* 1984; **102**: 527–532.

64 Savage S, Estacio RO, Jeffers B, *et al.* Urinary albumin excretion as a predictor of diabetic retinopathy, neuropathy and cardiovascular disease in NIDDM. *Diabetes Care* 1996; **19**: 1243–1248.

65 Hutchinson A, McIntosh A, Peters J, et al. Clinical Guidelines for Type 2 Diabetes: Diabetic retinopathy: Early management and screening. Sheffield: ScHARR, University of Sheffield, 2001. Online: http://www.shef.ac.uk/guidelines/

66 NICE Guideline Development Group and Recommend-ations Panel. *Inherited Clinical Guideline E. Management of type 2 Diabetes: Retinopathy – screening and early management.* London: NHS National Institute for Clinical Excellence, 2002. Online: http://www.nice.org.uk

67 NICE Guideline Development Group and Recommendations Panel. *Inherited Clinical Guideline F. Management of Type 2 Diabetes: Renal disease – prevention and early management.* London: NHS National Institute for Clinical Excellence, 2002. Online: http://www.nice.org.uk

68 MacLeod JM, Lutale J, Marshall SM. Albumin excretion and vascular deaths in NIDDM. *Diabetologia* 1995; **38**: 610–616.

69 Dinneen SF, Gerstein HC. The association of microalbuminuria and mortality in non-insulin-dependent diabetes mellitus. *Arch Int Med* 1997; **157**: 1413–1418.

70 American Diabetes Association: Position Statement. Diabetes nephropathy. *Diabetes Care* 2003; **26**(Suppl. 1): S94–S98.

71 Levene LS, McNally PG, Fraser RC, *et al. What is the Prevalence of Microalbuminuria in Patients with Diabetes in the Community?* Abstract presented to Diabetes UK 2002 professional conference.

72 Parving H-H, Lehnert H, Brochner-Mortensen J, *et al.* The effect of irbesartan on the development of diabetic nephropathy in patients with type 2 diabetes. *N Engl J Med* 2001; **345**: 870–878.

73 Brenner BM, Cooper ME, de Zeeuw D, *et al.* Effects of losartan on renal and cardiovascular outcomes in patients with type 2 diabetes and nephropathy. *N Engl J Med* 2001; **345**: 861–869.

74 Lewis EJ, Hunisicker LG, Clarke WR, *et al.* Renoprotective effect of the angiotensin-receptor antagonist irbesartan in patients with nephropathy due to type 2 diabetes. *N Engl J Med* 2001; **345**: 851–860.

75 Macleod AF. Diabetic neuropathy. *Medicine* 1997; **25**: 36–38.

76 Ralph D, McNicholas T for the Erectile Dysfunction Alliance. UK management guidelines for erectile dysfunction. *BMJ* 2000; **321**: 409–503.

CHAPTER NINE

Cardiovascular Disease Risk and Type 2 Diabetes

Cardiovascular disease (CVD) is a very significant cause of morbidity and mortality in patients with type 2 diabetes. The importance of reducing cardiovascular risk, one of the main aims of diabetic care, is a recurrent theme throughout this book, as reflected in the suggested protocol for the periodic review. The 'double whammy' of an increased prevalence of both type 2 diabetes and CHD in Indo-Asians indicates the need to correct vigorously the adverse cardiovascular risk factors in any vulnerable patient group. The purpose of this chapter is to provide an overview of the key concepts of cardiovascular risk reduction. More detailed discussions of the evaluation and intervention for individual risk factors can be found in Chapters 7 and 8.

Scale of the Problem

Overall, 5-year mortality in patients with type 2 diabetes increases two- to three-fold and age-adjusted life expectancy is reduced by 5–10 years compared to the general population,[1] with 58% of all mortality in type 2 diabetes cause by CVD alone.[2] Case mortality from myocardial infarction is greater in diabetics than in nondiabetics.

Evaluating Risk

Patients are at risk more from the combined impact of multiple cardiovascular risk factors than from a single risk factor. Usually, more than one of these risk factors will be found in an individual. Therefore, if a check reveals the presence of a cardiovascular risk factor, a search for the presence of other factors is necessary. A selection of charts and computer programs (e.g., the new Sheffield tables,[3] New Zealand tables[4] and joint British societies' charts and computer program for cardiovascular risk[5]) are all readily available to calculate the risk of cardiovascular outcomes for given combinations of clinical variables and to assess the impact of relevant interventions. These calculators are based upon data from the predominately Caucasian Framingham populations (which did not have a large number of individuals with diabetes) in the USA and are reasonably accurate predictors of CHD and CVD risk in a Caucasian UK population;[6] however, they underestimate risk in certain other ethnic groups (such as Indo-Asians and Afro-Caribbeans)[7] and in individuals with a positive family history of CHD.[8] These groups probably possess additional inherited risk factors, such as increased lipoprotein(a) levels in Indo-Asians, which could become more active when the cluster of conventional acquired cardiovascular factors are present.[9] This may explain why many studies show a steeper increased risk of developing CHD with increased total cholesterol in type 2 diabetics than in the nondiabetic population. Therefore, both professionals and patients need to accept the limitations of the above risk calculators in some patient groups.

Nevertheless, there is a practical need to undertake some form of risk assessment to guide management in dealing with targets, thresholds and the impact of interventions. For assessment purposes, the recently published National Clinical Guidelines for type 2 diabetes recommends an annual estimate of 10-year coronary event risk in people without manifest CVD and the division of all patients into higher and lower 10-year coronary event risk groups,[10,11] as defined in *Table 9.1*. Although 10 years appears now to be the accepted duration for vascular risk evaluation, it is less helpful in assessing risk in younger patients whose 'impending' event is likely to occur more than 10 years into the future. A major vascular event is calamitous whenever it actually occurs. For a young high-risk patient, interventions to influence events long into the future may provide few short-term gains, but may result in considerable benefit overall to that individual's health over a much greater potential lifespan. Thus, the allocation of individuals into the lower 10-year coronary event risk group could be considered arbitrary, as all type 2 diabetics have a high lifetime risk of developing vascular disease (see Chapter 3) and are likely to benefit over their lifetime from appropriate effective interventions to reduce that risk.

Table 9.1. Definitions of higher and lower 10-year coronary event risk

Stratification of risk	Definitions
Higher	Cardiovascular disease manifest (coronary heart disease, stroke or peripheral vascular disease) *or* 10-year coronary event risk is assessed as above 15%
Lower	Cardiovascular disease not manifest, *or* 10-year coronary event risk is assessed as 15% or below

Interventions to Reduce Cardiovascular Risk

Setting targets: an overview and practical considerations

Reducing cardiovascular risk (a real endpoint for patients) involves undertaking interventions to change reversible risk factors that are not real diseases in themselves for patients, but that are intermediates in the disease process. The rationale for the appropriate assessment of any intervention that reduces a risk factor is the decreased probability of a real endpoint happening to the patient: death or an event with real morbidity (such as a complication).

Two recent articles in the same issue of the *British Medical Journal* provide considerable food for thought as to the benefits of striving to achieve the targets advised by expert bodies.

In the first, Winocour[12] sounded a cautionary note, arguing that current targets (that started as a mean) were achieved in only 50–70% of research studies, and that to attain these targets involved polypharmacy, which may lead to reduced patient compliance. Furthermore, clinical guidelines may fail to take account of the drop-out rates in research studies. Starting with the typical cardiovascular risk profile of many patients with type 2 diabetes, professionals who aim to achieve the recommended targets may prescribe simultaneously two hypoglycaemic agents, three antihypertensive agents, one hypolipidaemic agent and aspirin: a total of seven

NSF
4

drugs, not including prescriptions for other medical problems. Is it any wonder that such a regimen is unacceptable to many patients? The logical conclusion to this argument is that, rather than the inflexible pursuit of several simultaneous 'tough' targets, it is surely reasonable in some cases to set pragmatic individualised targets, in full collaboration with the patient, with the main aim of improving the adverse measurement of each component. Two of Winocour's suggested alternative targets are given in *Table 9.2*. Readers may wish to bear these in mind, especially while reading the subsections on glycated haemoglobin and blood pressure in Chapter 8.

In the second article, Law and Wald proposed that we should regard variables, such as blood pressure, serum cholesterol and BMI (discussed below), as having a dose–response relationship with the diseases that they 'cause'.[13] They went on to argue 'that a given change in the variables reduces the risk of disease by a constant proportion of the existing risk irrespective of the starting level of the variable or existing risk.' They concluded that a patient's overall absolute level of risk, not the level of the risk factors, should determine the threshold for intervention. If a patient is assessed as carrying a high level of risk, intervention should aim for large changes in all the reversible risk factors together.[13] This approach appears to be supported by the findings of the MRC/BHF Heart Protection Study, which found benefit for high-risk patients from treatment with a statin, irrespective of the pretreatment cholesterol level.[14]

Perhaps the key messages to take from these articles are that:

- Targets should be set at a realistic and achievable level for the individual patient;
- All treatable risk factors should be attacked in patients identified as 'high risk';
- Any improvement in a risk factor is of benefit, whatever the starting point.

Table 9.2. Targets for certain measurable components of diabetic care[12]

Component	Current recommendation	Alternative recommendation	
		For an individual	For the clinic
HbA1c	6.5–7.5%	6.5% within 3 years of diagnosis, if no complications,on diet	50% <7.5%
		8% at 5 years after diagnosis, if complications	Reduction in clinic mean by 10–20%
		9% in insulin-treated obese	
Blood pressure (mmHg)	130–140/80–85	160/95 if aged >75 years	140/90 in 40% of treated patients
		150/90 if ischaemic heart disease, microalbuminuria, dyslipidaemia or smoker	160/95 in 75% of treated patients
		Reduce by 10–20%	Shift clinic mean by 10–20%

Risk factors: 'conventional' targets

Realistically, we cannot always determine accurately absolute risk and we may need to think about what levels of individual reversible risk factors confer increased risk, turning to the endpoint targets so beloved by expert bodies and those who seek to monitor our performance (see Chapter 8 for more detailed discussion):

- Smoking target – cessation;
- Blood pressure target – 130–140/80mmHg;
- Glycaemic control target – HbA1c less than 7.0%.
- Serum lipids target – below the level of increased CHD risk;
- Obesity target – BMI less than $25kg/m^2$ in men and $24kg/m^2$ in women, with no central obesity;
- Exercise target – reduce sedentary lifestyle as appropriate (see Chapter 8).

By tackling serum lipids, obesity and exercise, insulin resistance can be reduced (see Chapter 3). The UKPDS provided evidence that tight glycaemic control reduces both microvascular and macrovascular (such as cardiac) complications.[15-18] Further evidence is required to clarify whether achieving good glycaemic control primarily by reducing insulin resistance will reduce cardiovascular risk further.

Planning intervention

At all contacts with a type 2 diabetic patient, and especially at the periodic review, the professional needs to consider pragmatically what intervention(s) may be undertaken. Some success in reducing several risk factors collectively may be more helpful and acceptable to the patient than an obsessive quest to reduce a single factor to a tight target level.

Drug therapies are important, but should complement, not replace, appropriate health education, which requires time and skill (see Chapter 12). Diabetic patients have a key role in the management of their disease (see Chapters 5 and 12) and may require guidance and support to achieve their optimal lifestyle.

NSF
3

Aspirin

Secondary prevention

There is a clear consensus to prescribe 75mg aspirin daily in people with manifest CVD.

Primary prevention

The current recommendations by the National Clinical Guidelines for type 2 diabetes is to offer 75mg aspirin daily to people with a 10-year coronary event risk of greater than 15%, with the proviso that the systolic blood pressure be reduced to 145mmHg or below prior to starting aspirin therapy.[11]

The ADA's latest recommendations state that low-dose aspirin should be 'considered' in diabetics aged over 40 years with at least one of the following risk factors for a cardiovascular event:[19]

- Family history of CHD;
- Cigarette smoking;
- Hypertension;
- Obesity (BMI greater than 27.3 in women; greater than 27.8 in men);
- Albuminuria (micro- or macro-);
- Adverse lipid profile.

Diabetes UK recommends that, as well as the above, the following risk factors in diabetics *may* warrant aspirin treatment:[20]

- Indo-Asian origin;
- The presence of diabetic retinopathy.

Any prescribing of aspirin should be according to the recognised cautions and contraindications given in the BNF (Sections 2.9 and 4.7.1).[21] These include:

- Aspirin allergy;
- Bleeding tendency;
- Concurrent anticoagulant therapy;
- Recent gastrointestinal bleeding;
- Clinically active hepatic disease;
- Children under the age of 16 years.

Key Points in this Chapter

- Often more than one cardiovascular risk factor is present, and their combined impact is more devastating than any single factor.
- Cardiac risk calculators are useful, but can underestimate risk in Indo-Asians and those with a positive family history.
- Targets should be set at a realistic and achievable level for the individual patient.
- All treatable risk factors should be attacked in patients identified as 'high risk'.
- Any improvement in a risk factor is of benefit, whatever the starting point.

REFERENCES

1 Panzram G. Mortality and survival in Type 2 (non-insulin dependent) diabetes mellitus. *Diabetologia* 1987; **30**: 123–131.

2 Davies MJ, Burden AC, Burden ML. Screening for type 2: increasing evidence that it is necessary. Part 1: Should it be done? *Practical Diabetes Int* 1997; **14**: 162–164.

3 Wallis EJ, Ramsay LE, Haq IU, *et al.* Coronary and cardiovascular risk estimation for primary prevention: validation of a new Sheffield table in the 1995 Scottish health survey population. *BMJ* 2000; **320**: 671–676.

4 Dyslipidaemia Advisory Group on behalf of the scientific committee of the National Heart Foundation of New Zealand. National Heart Foundation guidelines for the assessment and management of dyslipidaemia. *NZ Med J* 1996; **109**: 224–232.

5. British Hypertension Society. Online: http://www.hyp.ac.uk/bhs/resources/guidelines.htm

6 Hingorani AD, Vallance P. A simple computer program for guiding management of cardiovascular risk factors and prescribing. *BMJ* 1999; **318**: 101–105.

7 Cappuccio FP, Oakeshott P, Strazzullo P, *et al.* Application of Framingham risk estimates to ethnic minorities in United Kingdom and implications for primary prevention of heart disease in general practice: cross-sectional population based study. *BMJ* 2002; **325**: 1271–1276.

8 Silberberg J, Wlodarczyk J, Fryer J, *et al.* Risk associated with various definitions of family history of coronary artery disease. The Newcastle family history study II. *Am J Epidemiol* 1998; **147**: 1133–1139.

9 Lawrence IG, McNally PG. Heart disease in Asian people with diabetes. *Practical Diabetes Int* 2001; **18**: 192–196.

10 McIntosh A, Hutchinson A, Feder G, *et al. Clinical Guidelines and Evidence Review for Type 2 Diabetes: Lipids management.* Sheffield: ScHARR, University of Sheffield, 2002. Online: http://shef.ac.uk/guidelines

11 Hutchinson A, McIntosh A, Griffiths CJ, *et al. Clinical Guidelines and Evidence Review for Type 2 Diabetes: Blood pressure management.* Sheffield: ScHARR, University of Sheffield, 2002. Online: http://shef.ac.uk/guidelines

12 Winocour PH. Effective diabetes care: a need for realistic targets. *BMJ* 2002; **324**: 1577–1580.

13 Law MR, Wald NJ. Risk factor thresholds: their existence under scrutiny. *BMJ* 2002; **324**: 1370–1376.

14 Collins R, Armitage J, Parish S, *et al.* for the Heart Protection Study Collaborative Group. MRC/BHF Heart Protection Study of cholesterol lowering with simvastatin in 20,536 high-risk individuals: a randomised placebo-controlled trial. *Lancet* 2002; **360**: 7–22.

15 UK Prospective Diabetes Study Group. Tight blood pressure control and risk of macro vascular and micro vascular complications in type 2 diabetes: UKPDS 38. *BMJ* 1998; **317**: 703–712.

16 UK Prospective Diabetes Study Group. Intensive blood-glucose control with sulphonylureas or insulin compared with conventional treatment and risk of complications in patients with type 2 diabetes (UKPDS 33). *Lancet* 1998; **352**: 837–853.

17 UK Prospective Diabetes Study Group. Effect of intensive blood-glucose control with metformin on complications in overweight patients with type 2 diabetes (UKPDS 34). *Lancet* 1998; **352**: 854–865

18 Stratton IM, Adler AI, Neil HAW, *et al.* Association of glycaemia with macrovascular and microvascular complications of type 2 diabetes (UKPDS 35): prospective observational study. *BMJ* 2000; **321**: 405–412.

19 American Diabetes Association. Position Statement: aspirin therapy in diabetes. *Diabetes Care* 2003; **26** (Suppl. 1): S87–S88

20 Diabetes UK. Online: http://www.diabetes.org.uk

21 Joint Formulary Committee. *British National Formulary 44*. London: British Medical Association and Royal Pharmaceutical Society of Great Britain, 2002.

CHAPTER TEN

Emergencies

Metabolic Emergencies

Hypoglycaemia

Definition

Hypoglycaemia is an abnormally low blood glucose level that leads to symptoms of sympathetic nervous system stimulation or of central nervous system dysfunction.

Causes

The causes of hypoglycaemia in patients with type 2 diabetes are:

- Drug induced, such as by insulin, sulphonylureas, repaglinide, alcohol;
- Missed or small meal;
- Unplanned exercise;
- Combination of the above.

Interventions

The interventions include:

- *Prevention* by education of the patient and close family members on the warning symptoms; timing of medication, meals and physical activity; the need to always carry identification and/or a warning card or bracelet and 'instant carbohydrate'.
- *Confirm* by testing blood glucose, ideally using an accurate blood glucose machine.
- *Immediate correction* of low blood glucose – if conscious and co-operative, use 'instant carbohydrate'; otherwise inject glucagon (ensure the family has a device and the instructions).
- If a patient suffers from repeated hypoglycaemia, an *evaluation* of diet, lifestyle and drug treatment, followed by appropriate adjustments, is necessary (see Chapters 7 and 8 for more details).

Intercurrent illness

The stress of illness can produce transient insulin resistance and worsen glycaemic control, and so requires more frequent monitoring of blood or urine glucose. Patients treated with oral hypoglycaemic drugs or diet alone may need a temporary increase in their glucose lowering treatment, either by using a higher dose of existing treatment and/or by by introducing a new agent (usually insulin). At the same time, an adequate fluid and calorific intake must be maintained, especially if the patient is vomiting. Hospital admission may be necessary more often in diabetics to treat infection and/or correct dehydration.

Hyperosmolar nonketotic hyperglycaemic coma

The syndrome hyperosmolar nonketotic hyperglycaemic coma (HONK) is a complication of type 2 diabetes and is characterised by hyperglycaemia, extreme dehydration and hyperosmolar plasma, and leads to impaired consciousness. It has a very high mortality rate, particularly in frail and/or socially isolated elderly patients. Hyperglycaemia accompanied by an inadequate fluid intake leads to extreme dehydration, a situation that can be triggered by a co-existing acute infection. Treatment is immediate hospital admission to correct fluid balance and biochemistry.

Vascular Emergencies

Myocardial infarction

Not only are type 2 diabetics at increased risk of suffering a coronary heart event, but also the presentation may be atypical, and thus delay their receiving appropriate medical care. It is not infrequent for elderly diabetics to suffer no chest pain during an infarct. The only clues may be an ill patient, with some degree of cardiac dysfunction (abnormal pulse, hypotensive or signs of heart failure) and hyperglycaemia. Acute hospital admission may be needed to confirm diagnosis or to deal with more complex management problems and social circumstances.

Following an acute myocardial infarction (MI), patients with diabetes should be considered for intensive insulin treatment (currently under evaluation, but with promising results), as well as for the standard therapies of thrombolysis, beta blockers, antiplatelet therapy (aspirin, with the possible addition of clopidogrel) and ACE inhibitors (especially if there is any evidence of left ventricular dysfunction). Although all these therapies have their own side effects, the increased mortality of MI and the further risk of a second event justify a more aggressive approach in patients with diabetics.

Lower limb problems

Evaluation and intervention are discussed in detail in Chapter 8. A loss of skin integrity that leads to an ulcer or gangrene is a potential emergency. Prevention and, if this fails, prompt appropriate management are essential to minimise any permanent damage or limb loss.

Vitreous haemorrhage

Vitreous haemorrhage arises usually from retinal new vessels. Chapter 8 provides further details on how to detect new vessels. The patient often presents with acute visual loss. Immediate referral to a hospital ophthalmologist is indicated.

Cerebrovascular disease

Cerebrovascular disease is the second most common cause of death in patients with type 2 diabetes and can cause a range of devastating deficits:

- *Hemiplegia* is usually the result of atheromatous cerebrovascular disease, but it can be a rare transient manifestation of hypoglycaemia in patients on insulin;
- Other *reversible focal neurological deficits* also usually result from atheromatous cerebrovascular disease, but can occur in the rare HONK discussed above;

- *Convulsions* may result from structural cerebral damage caused by cerebrovascular disease, but can be triggered by hyperglycaemia if there is hyperosmolarity in susceptible patients;
- *Cognitive impairment* may result from atherosclerotic dementia, but hyperglycaemia is also thought to produce psychological dysfunction. Better glycaemic control may improve cognition.

In addition to hypertension and increasing age, atrial fibrillation has been identified by the UKPDS as a major risk factor for stroke in patients with type 2 diabetes.[1] As well as vigorous correction of other risk factors (optimising blood pressure and lipid profile, smoke cessation), anticoagulation should be considered, with aspirin as an alternative if anticoagulation is either contraindicated or unsuitable. Guidance on the optimal management of atrial fibrillation can be found in *Clinical Evidence*.[2]

Key Point of this Chapter

- Prompt recognition and effective intervention reduce the impact of metabolic and vascular emergencies.

REFERENCES

1   Davies TME, Millns H, Stratton IM, *et al.* Risk factors for stroke in non-insulin dependent diabetes mellitus: UKPDS 29. *Arch Intern Med* 1999; **159**: 1097–1103.

2   Lip GYH, Kamath S, Freestone B. Acute atrial fibrillation. *Clin Evid* 2003; **8**. Online (free to NHS staff via the National Electronic Library of Health): http://www.nelh.nhs.uk/clinical_evidence.asp

CHAPTER ELEVEN

Special Problems and Circumstances

Psychological Health in Patients with Diabetes

Individuals with a chronic disease such as diabetes are more vulnerable to a range of psychological and psychiatric disorders. Depression and anxiety are more common in diabetics than in the general population. The presence of complications further lowers the quality of life and increases the likelihood of depression. The interaction between mental health and diabetes can lead to a vicious cycle of worsening diabetic management and mental illness.

From diagnosis, health care professionals and carers can play an important role in the mental health of diabetics:

- By providing adequate psychological support to enable patients to come to terms with their diabetes and to take increasing control of their disease, one of the aims of care (see Chapter 5). Diabetes can cause psychological distress, separate from mental illness.
- By early recognition and appropriate management of mental illness, which can affect diabetic care adversely. Involvement of the local mental health team or liaison psychiatrist may be necessary. Depression with biological features usually requires pharmacological therapy, preferably with a selective serotonin reuptake inhibitor (SSRI), which may improve glycaemic control.[1]
- By recognising the full range of nonmedical (e.g., social, financial) factors than can affect patients and by accepting that in the patients' minds these may have precedence over diabetes and other medical problems – solving other problems may be the most effective way to improve both diabetic and mental health.

Cognitive behaviour therapy (CBT; see also Chapter 12) is also useful in treating depression, but is less effective in diabetic patients with complications.[2]

Driving

Legal provisions

The Road Traffic Acts require that all diabetics treated other than by diet alone report their condition to the licensing centre (DVLA Drivers' Medical Unit, Longview Road, Morriston, Swansea SA99 1TU). Professionals should document giving this advice in the patients' records for medico-legal reasons.[3] The patient must inform the DVLA if any problems or diabetic complications develop that may affect the safety of driving. The visual standards are the same as for nondiabetics: a corrected Snellen chart visual acuity of 6/12 and a visual field of at least 120° in the horizontal axis and at least 20° in the vertical axis.

Group I (ordinary) licence holders and applicants treated with insulin must demonstrate satisfactory control, recognise the warning symptoms of hypoglycaemia, and not suffer from a relevant disability. They are granted a one-, two- or three-year licence. On renewal they are required to make a self-declaration that may lead to medical enquiries. Those treated with diet and tablets or diet alone are permitted to hold a licence valid to 70 years of age, subject to the conditions given above and the need to report any change to insulin treatment.

Since 1st April 1991, diabetic patients on insulin have been banned from applying for and renewing thereafter a *Group 2* (bus, coach and large goods vehicle driver) licence. Diabetics on diet alone or diet and tablet treatment are permitted to hold a Group 2 licence, subject to the absence of any relevant disability and to not being on insulin.

Insulin is a drug within the meaning of the Road Traffic Act 1988, and a driver 'in control of a motor vehicle' with symptoms of hypoglycaemia runs the risk of being charged with driving under the influence of drugs.

Insurance

Valid car insurance requires that drivers inform their insurance companies at the time of diagnosis (irrespective of whether control is by diet alone, oral medication or insulin). Some insurance companies may charge higher premiums and it is worthwhile shopping around for the most competitive quote. Diabetes UK has a motor insurance quote line on 0800 731 7432, but, although sympathetic to people with diabetes, they may not always be the cheapest.

Medical aspects

Medical aspects are:[3]

- *Hypoglycaemia* can impair driving performance significantly. Diabetic drivers should aim always to prevent hypoglycaemia. If this fails, and the symptoms of hypoglycaemia present, prompt treatment with emergency sugar is crucial.
- *Visual problems* arise usually from either retinopathy or cataract. As well as incorrectable deterioration of visual acuity, loss of peripheral visual field through widespread ablative retinal photocoagulation may result in loss of fitness to drive.
- Neurological and/or vascular deficit may result in severe *damage to the feet* (leading to ulcers, or even amputation), and so also results in loss of fitness to drive.
- *Arterial disease* may result in cardiovascular and/or cerebrovascular disability, which affect fitness to drive.

'Have Diabetes, Can Travel'

Patients with type 2 diabetes do and should travel. They should observe the same precautions as the rest of the population, but also they should make their own special arrangements to reduce the risk of diabetic complications and emergencies. Constant perfect glycaemic control is not an absolute necessity, but the extremes of hypoglycaemia and hyperglycaemia should be avoided. Pre-travel planning is essential and should involve obtaining essential information, ensuring current optimal diabetic management and having in place all the necessary arrangements. Health care professionals and organisations, such as Diabetes UK[4] and the Tayside Regional Diabetes Network,[5] can provide useful information.

Vaccinations

Diabetics are advised to have the necessary vaccinations well in advance of departure, as these may cause a transient disturbance of glycaemic control.

Packing

Diabetics should pack and carry sufficient and suitably packed supplies of their medication (including either glucagon or glucose tablets to treat hypoglycaemia), and the documentation for their trip. Any glass items should be wrapped carefully in socks or placed between soft clothing during transport. If flying, then medication, supplies and documentation should be packed in carry-on luggage, rather than in checked or stowed baggage. Extra quantities should be taken in case of delays, mishaps or if further supplies are unlikely to be available at the destination.

Insulin should be kept out of direct sunlight and should always be kept cool, either in a cool bag or some form of cool storage, although open insulin vials retain their potency at temperate room temperatures for up to one month. Insulin should *not* be kept in car glove compartments (too hot) or in checked luggage (too cold).

Prescription medications should be kept in their original containers, and other items (such as syringes, alcohol swabs and test strips) should be packed in plastic bags with zipper-type seals.

Medication

In a few countries insulin is not available in U100 strength, but in U40. If patients switch to U40 insulin abroad, to ensure the correct dose they should also use U40 syringes and so avoid any mixture with U100.

Documentation

Patients should wear or carry some form of medical identification, such as a bracelet or necklace. In this period of heightened concerns about travel security, diabetic travellers should carry a practice- or hospital-headed letter from their doctor or nurse that lists their medical problems, medication and supplies, and confirms that their medication and devices are required and appropriate for their personal therapeutic needs. This letter could also be useful if seeking medical attention abroad.

Insurance

It is prudent to obtain adequate travel insurance and to carry the necessary sickness insurance forms in case of illness abroad. It is important to check that 'pre-existing conditions' are not excluded.

Medical attention is officially free in all European Union countries for UK residents, provided the patient has obtained an E111 certificate (from a Post Office) before departure to prove eligibility for treatment. However, treatment under the E111 scheme may not be adequate for diabetes. Diabetes UK can advise.[4]

Treatment regimes

Travelling across time zones and eating different foods at unpredictable times both require adjustment of treatment regimes, particularly if on insulin. Some of the principles used for diabetics who observe fasting during Ramadan may apply (see Chapter 7). In aiming to avoid hypoglycaemia or marked hyperglycaemia, diabetics may be permitted to run their blood sugars slightly higher, reduce the quantity of basal insulin to the dose necessary to keep blood sugars 'ticking over' and take rapid-acting insulin with meals. High temperatures can increase insulin absorption. This should be taken into account when travelling or exercising in hot climates. Thus, a reduction in the insulin dose may be indicated.

If on oral medication, diabetics may wish to transfer to a shorter-acting sulphonylurea during the journey.

Diabetics should be advised never to stop insulin and/or oral hypoglycaemic medication, even if unable to take solid foods. They should discuss managing vomiting and diarrhoea with their diabetes team prior to departure, but they should seek local medical help if symptoms persist or if they become ill.

Other precautions

It is advisable to take a good supply of food and drink for delays, but not to ask for a 'diabetic meal' from the airline as these often contain no carbohydrate. Drinking only bottled water, avoiding salads and being careful about hygiene levels in restaurants are sensible precautions.

Diabetics need to take on holiday comfortable, well-fitting shoes in case their feet swell in hot weather. They must beware of going barefoot, particularly on hot sand.

As with nondiabetic travellers, suitable emergency medication should be carried, if appropriate.

Cultural Aspects of Diabetes Care

Mary MacKinnon's book covers this area well and in greater detail.[6] An understanding of different cultures by professionals helps to ensure that suitable advice is given, and offence and misunderstandings are avoided, where possible.

General points

- There are considerable differences and variations in customs, health beliefs, etiquettes and diet, even within the same region.
- In contrast to the English sequence of 'vision, hearing and touch', other cultures may prefer the sequence of 'touch, hearing and vision'.
- If English is not the patient's first language, the professional must be patient.
- Afro-Asian patients may prefer to be examined by a professional of the same gender.
- The role of other members of the family and their community may be important.
- Smoking is quite common among Hindus, Muslims and Bangladeshis.
- Even though alcohol is prohibited by some religions, its consumption, and even abuse, may still occur.
- Many Afro-Asian diabetics use various types of traditional and/or herbal medicines regularly, even if they are taking conventional therapeutic medicines. Karela or guard is a recognised insulin-like substance.
- In Afro-Asian culture, a greater emphasis is placed on physical symptoms than on psychological ones, and there may be a greater expectation upon the doctor to make a diagnosis without a full assessment and to provide a prescription rather than advice.
- Many Asians may feel that the diagnosis of diabetes is a stigma and consider the disease to be contagious.

Specific examples

Islam

Ramadan is discussed at the end of Chapter 7. Muslims are forbidden strictly to drink alcohol and to eat pork. Alternatives to porcine insulin and to tablets or capsules that contain gelatine must be provided.

Hinduism

There are many strands of Hinduism. Hindu festivals involve the exchange of sweets, which may play havoc with glycaemic control. Many Hindus are vegetarian and can consume food with a high fat content.

Key Points of this Chapter

- Diabetics are more vulnerable to anxiety and depression.
- Legal and medical considerations affect driving by diabetics.
- Additional care will reduce the risks of travel problems in diabetics.
- There are considerable differences and variations in customs, health beliefs, etiquettes and diet among different cultures. The professional must be aware of these to reduce offence and misunderstandings.

REFERENCES

1 Lustman PJ, Freedland KE, Griffith LS, *et al.* Flouxetine for depression in diabetes: a randomized double-blind placebo-controlled trial. *Diabetes Care* 2000; **236**: 618–623.

2 Lustman PJ, Griffith LS, Freedland KE, *et al.* Cognitive behaviour therapy for depression in type 2 diabetes mellitus. A randomized, controlled trial. *Ann Intern Med* 1988; **129**: 613–621.

3 Keen H. Diabetes mellitus. In: Taylor JF (Ed). *Medical Aspects of Fitness to Drive*. 5th Edn. London: The Medical Commission on Accident Prevention, 1995.

4 Diabetes UK. Careline contactable by telephone. 020 7424 1030 (Weekdays 9AM to 5PM). Online: http://www.diabetes.org.uk

5 Tayside Regional Diabetes Network, Online: http://www.diabetes-healthnet.ac.uk/

6 MacKinnon M. *Providing Diabetes Care in General Practice: A Practical Guide for the Primary Care Team.* 4th Edn. London: Class Publishing, 2002.

CHAPTER TWELVE

Patient Education and Lifestyle Modification

NSF 3

Type 2 diabetes is an excellent example of a chronic medical condition in which patients are the key players in their future well-being. Health care professionals must never forget that the patients 'own' their disease and play a crucial role in their own glycaemic control, well-being and prevention of complications. One of the professional's key roles is to provide advice and support, with the aim of promoting self-care. Health education begins at diagnosis and each subsequent professional encounter with the type 2 diabetic patient is an opportunity for further education. Frequently, this is more than merely imparting information. To improve a less than optimal lifestyle is often at the centre of disease prevention and management, as discussed in previous chapters. Primary care professionals trained to take a 'patient-centred' approach when delivering lifestyle interventions are more likely than those in secondary care to improve patient satisfaction and knowledge.[1] As mentioned in previous chapters, professionals need to be aware that other factors may affect their patients and that, until these issues are addressed, changes and improved care will be delayed and less likely to result.

A Personal View

Many GPs and practice nurses lack both the time and skills to provide effective health education. And yet, to provide suitable advice is one of the components of management (termed RAPRIO, see Chapter 6). Professionals do attempt to provide short bursts of 'health education' in many of their consultations that deal with chronic disease. Over a long period, such as a month or year, the total time devoted to all of these interventions is considerable. So why not do it well? On rare occasions, professionals have changed patients' behaviours by a single piece of advice. More frequent occurrences of such outcomes would both benefit patients and increase professionals' job satisfaction. How can we increase the 'success' rate?

Every professional can conjure up a list of the 'usual suspects', who consult regularly, whose chronic problems are caused or exacerbated by their poor lifestyle and who remain impervious to suggestions to modify their behaviour, but who eternally expect the professional to provide the nonexistent 'miracle cure'. Improving lifestyle to reduce vascular risk in these individuals is a difficult challenge.

Patients often know more than is credited to them. The main aim of health education is more often to change behaviour than to give information. This requires an approach that is not didactic, but that draws upon the experience of educationalists and psychologists.

The author has found it useful to draw upon four overlapping concepts in a simplistic way to guide educational interventions within the consultation:
- effective consultation technique;
- the educational triangle;

- the trans-theoretical model of change;
- cognitive behaviour therapy, problem solving and motivational approaches.

Effective consultation technique

Most GPs, particularly those involved in training, are aware of the extensive literature on the con-sultation process. It is far beyond the scope of this book to discuss these ideas in any depth and there are many different consultation models, but health professionals should aim to use good effective consultation behaviours in all patient contacts, without slighting the necessary clinical content. The author found a recent overview useful.[2] In the consultation, professionals should maintain a broader focus on physical, emotional and social factors, and they should involve patients in decisions in a way that is both appropriate and effective for the patient and the professional.

One model (among many) for the medical encounter consists of three 'functions':

- *Building the relationship* includes active listening without interruption and responding to issues raised by patients (especially emotional ones);
- *Defining the problem(s)* includes eliciting the patient's agenda, considering other factors and 'sharing' an understanding of the diagnosis;
- *Agreeing a management plan* includes providing information and appropriate reassurance, making links between the problem's presentation and a diagnosis, and negotiating a man-agement plan and behaviour change.

Professionals are more likely to carry out these functions within their consultations if they deploy the skills of good communication and effective problem solving. The Gask and Usherwood article[2] provides a helpful list of concepts and techniques, and John Launer's book provides an interesting and practical approach to the consultation in primary care.[3]

Educational triangle

GP trainers will recall the established triad of aims, methods and assessment, which can be applied also to patient education:

- *Aims* can be to address any combination of knowledge, skill or attitude 'needs', as agreed by the learner and the provider;
- *Methods* may involve a range of activities from one-on-one to groups to printed and video literature (see later in this chapter);
- *Assessment* is formative and on-going, identifying needs and monitoring progress towards targets.

Trans-theoretical model of change

The likelihood of changing various health-related behaviours, such as smoking, alcohol con-sumption, diet and exercise, may be related to the patient's position in the trans-theoretical model of change.[4,5] Individuals who are at the *pre-contemplation* stage are not interested in change. Those at the *contemplation* stage are thinking about change, and can be guided through the stages of *preparing to change, making the change* and *maintaining the change,* hopefully with the outcome of a safer or healthier behaviour. Relapses can occur, but, if these are recognised, patients can be guided back into the change cycle. Various triggers may cause patients to move from being unwilling to one of thinking about change. This process may include realising that they are susceptible, that the problem is connected to their current behav-iour and that the benefits of change outweigh the risks and/or disadvantages.

Cognitive behaviour therapy, problem solving and motivational approaches

Cognitive behaviour therapy (CBT) refers to a group of psychological treatments that include behaviour therapy, behaviour modification and cognitive therapy in various combinations. *Behaviour approaches* aim to change behaviour, both as a therapeutic aim in its own right, and to produce other symptomatic improvements. *Cognitive approaches* explore how cognition mediates feelings and behaviour. Therapy aims to identify maladaptive thought patterns and to teach the patient to recognise and challenge these. In practice, therapists combine both approaches.[6]

CBT has a wide range of established clinical applications, especially for mental health problems, such as depression, panic disorder and post-traumatic stress disorder.[7] However, there is now an increasing interest in using CBT techniques to modify other behaviours – psychotherapists do not have a monopoly in this area. GPs and nurses can be trained easily to undertake brief, focussed CBT interventions that are more likely to be effective than the brief lecture of 'do this'. CBT interventions consist of three sequential steps (usually undertaken over several encounters):

1 *Baseline*, 'Where are you now?' The professional aims to identify the current state (behaviours, thoughts and feelings) of the patient in regard to condition and well-being. This information, particularly if elicited in a structured way, is important for later evaluation, for developing rapport and for assisting change by starting the process of goal setting.

2 *Outcome*, 'Where do you want to get to?' This requires patients to define their goals and aims to assist them towards their 'picture of health'. The professional helps the patient to explore the benefits of change, with attention to the expected gains (physical, psychological and cognitive). These may include greater autonomy. The grid in *Figure 12.1* is a possible technique for this exploration. Goal identification enables the patient and professional to know when the intervention is completed, and thus provides momentum for change.

3 *Process*, 'How are we going to get there?' Both patient and professional need to contribute to achieving the goals, with clearly defined responsibilities. The agreed plan of action may include various techniques, including problem solving, graded task setting (small manageable goals to generate greater self-confidence from success), visualisation, interpersonal 'coaching' and other educational techniques.

Applying CBT to the trans-theoretical model, the patient is at the contemplative stage when the outcome has moved away from the baseline.

	Benefits	Loses
No change		
Change		

Figure 12.1. Grid to help explore the benefits of change.

Changing Behaviour

Behavioural change is a personal process that can follow the above CBT sequence. The involved professional must have an understanding of and a respect for individuals, and strong 'interpersonal' skills (including being a good communicator). The professional should also be able to negotiate with patients some specific plans with clear goals that require concrete actions in small steps, to provide constructive feedback and to develop the patients' ability to learn from their lapses.

The professional's approach can start with employing effective consulting techniques to ensure good communication with the patient, adding motivational approaches and then going on to use CBT techniques. Those who seek to integrate these skills into their daily practice require training, practice and regular feedback.

Motivational behaviour influences lifestyle and is owned by the individual. One way of looking at motivation is to start by considering the components importance and confidence. *Importance* is made up of:

- Knowledge about the pros and cons of any behaviour;
- Concern (balance between too little and too much) about that behaviour.

Confidence is made up of:

- Self-esteem;
- Self-efficacy (belief in ability to act).

If both awareness of the importance of change and confidence to undertake it are sufficient, the individual is ready to change (this corresponds to the contemplative stage of the transtheoretical model).

Structured information gathering by professionals enable them to develop a greater understanding of the current situation: the constructs of the patient's motivation (importance of current behaviour and patient's self-confidence) and an awareness of what goals might be feasible. Simple questions can be asked to explore importance, along the lines of:

- 'How do you feel now, on a scale of 1 to 10?'
- 'On a scale of 1 to 10, how important is *xyz* to you?'
- 'What would have to happen before you would seriously consider change?'

and confidence, along the lines of:

- 'How confident, on a scale of 1 to 10, do you feel about being able to change *xyz*?'
- 'How can I help you to make that change?'
- 'How successful have you been in previous attempts – what went wrong?'

To identify and stimulate the patient's awareness of the need for change, the professional can use motivational 'linguistic patterns' to emphasise the benefits of change, such as 'As you begin eating more healthily and regularly, you will notice that your general well-being improves as your blood sugar becomes stable, and, because of this, you will have more energy.'

Where there is ambivalence, a useful exercise is to ask the patient to complete a grid, such as that in *Figure 12.1* (this can be done away from the consultation).

Ultimately, patients need to be 'enabled' to express concern about their current behaviour and the arguments for change, so that their 'decisional balance' is tipped towards action and, hence, the readiness to change.

In the domain of a psychological approach, the professional needs to be aware of the effects of secondary gain, control and emotional expression within the patient's illness behaviour. Most people know what is good for them and how to achieve it. Just as smoking-cessation interventions are ineffective when the 'benefits' to the patient of remaining a smoker are ignored, so too can some features be overlooked within the psychological management of physical conditions. An example is the patient who, after a row with his or her partner, sabotages some aspect of the diabetic programme (ignores diet, omits medication) to force the partner to take the roles of rescuer and consoler. This sabotage may be how a patient expresses anger, but it has negative health consequences. In contrast, healthy people under stress, who push themselves too far and risk adverse health, are not 'saboteurs'. The professional who is aware of these other features can challenge the patient and apply problem solving to help the patient take 'ownership' of his or her behaviour and to bring out into the open unconscious motives.

Putting Health Education into Practice for Patients with Diabetes

General principles of the process of health education

Whatever is done, good communication is essential. Many studies show a clear correlation between effective doctor–patient communication and improved patient health outcomes.[8] Some thought needs to be given as to how to understand and reach out to diabetics who do not speak English, such as elderly Indo-Asians, before undertaking any health education. Access to an interpreter and appropriate written material is helpful.

To construct an effective health education programme involves the following:

- The patient's *needs are identified and addressed*. As stated above, health education should be about more than increasing the patient's knowledge and skills (although this is essential for each patient to self-manage the disease); it should also be about helping the patient to modify lifestyle or behaviour. The content of any health education package should be geared to the time of and the need for its use.
- Where appropriate, the patient's *willingness and barriers to change are identified*. Thus, the professional needs to understand the patient's position on the trans-theoretical model of change discussed above and to be prepared to use CBT or other psychological techniques to help each patient move towards a readiness to change if this is feasible.
- The patient and the team *agree the aims of care* and the methods used to achieve these aims. These need to be realistic for each individual patient, respect the patient's autonomy, increase the patient's freedom of action and have perceived and sustained benefit. The professional contributes knowledge and skills to any discussion. Failure to agree will not change an unhealthy life style.
- Advice given is *based upon the evidence* and *appropriate* to the psychological and social circumstances of the patient.
- A clear *explanation about the importance and rationale* of any advice or intervention is given in terms that the patient understands clearly.
- *Expectations* of performance, by both the patient and/or professional, are *realistic* for that individual patient. Otherwise, disappointment is more likely than success, and the perceived failure is likely to result in poor compliance.
- All the involved professionals give similar and not contradictory advice, that is *stay 'on message'*, to use a currently fashionable political expression.
- *Prepare the patient for changes* as the need arises.

Specific topics of health education for diabetics and type of interventions

The curriculum of health education topics for a patient with diabetes is large, in depth, range and techniques to be used. In broad terms, these should include:

- Lifestyle – diet and alcohol consumption, smoking and exercise;
- Glycaemic control – self-monitoring and administration of therapy (e.g., insulin);
- Complications – foot care;
- Administration – prescriptions and follow-up.

The factual content of these areas is covered in depth in Chapters 7 and 8.

In their guidelines, SIGN[9] and, in particular detail, the University of Sheffield sponsored by NICE[10] reviewed the evidence for the effectiveness of different interventions on modifying the lifestyle of patients with diabetes. In 2003, NICE intends to issue a technology appraisal of patient education models for diabetes. The evidence is not always consistent and further work is required, but much research is in progress and the picture should become progressively clearer. The key recommendations are that patient education should be ongoing and that different approaches should be used until the best methods to achieve the desired outcomes for each patient are identified.

Evidence for the impact of various intervention approaches on specific diabetic topics

A brief summary of the evidence is given here:

- *Patient education in general.* The type of education provided seems less important than whether it is actually provided and received.
- *Knowledge and skills.* A variety of approaches have been shown to have inconsistent benefits, but none cause any decrease in patients' knowledge and skills.
- *Glycated haemoglobin.* No clear evidence indicates which educational approach works best.
- *Weight loss.* Different interventions can work, but their beneficial effects diminish over time.
- *Smoking cessation* (see Chapter 8 for a fuller discussion). Individual advice by a professional has a small but significant effect, increased by NRT and/or bupropion therapy.
- *Exercise and physical activity.* No trial-based evidence indicates the optimal method for promoting physical activity in the diabetic population. Evidence from nondiabetic populations supports using CBT skills, identifying the patient's position on the trans-theoretical model of change (both discussed above) and providing on-going support to maintain any behavioural change.[11]
- *Healthy eating.* Limited evidence indicates that assessment (using the trans-theoretical model of change) of readiness to change diet behaviour should be undertaken before giving dietary advice to diabetics. Dietary changes are more likely if psychological approaches are used.

What methods are available for delivering patient education?

The delivery of health education can use numerous methods. Primary care professionals may not use all of these methods regularly yet, but there may be scope to use some of their features routinely. The comments below summarise the evidence given in the University of Sheffield guidelines and some practical comments about their relevance to a primary care setting.

Didactic-based approach

The traditional didactic-based approach has little interaction, as the patient is a passive recipient of 'good advice'. Unfortunately, this approach will continue because most professionals are accustomed to using a didactic approach, other methods require more time and effort, and some patients just want to be told what they should do. Not surprisingly, there is no consistent evidence that this approach has a beneficial effect on glycaemic control or on weight loss.

Behaviour-modification approach

A behaviour-modification approach encompasses a broad range of strategies (as discussed above), is 'multi-faceted' and focuses mostly on diet and exercise. There is supporting evidence for a positive effect on weight reduction, but there is less evidence for improvements in glycaemic control and knowledge. With training, any health care professional can use psychological techniques effectively in a brief consultation.

Telephone-delivered education

A telephone-delivered education approach involves telephone follow-up by the professional to promote healthy behaviour and compliance with treatment, and to discuss any patient queries. There is very limited evidence for a possible improvement in glycated haemoglobin, but no evidence for a positive impact on either weight loss or knowledge. Telephone contact between patient and professional is used increasingly for queries and to adjust the management of on-going problems, if only to reduce the pressure on overstretched appointment systems. The advantages may be greater flexibility and convenience for both patient and professional, but even telephone consultations require time and cannot be combined with an examination or any nonverbal evaluation.

Group-management approach

The group-management approach promotes patient interaction within a group setting, and aims to change dietary and exercise habits, which should lead to improved glycaemic control. Again, evidence is very limited as to the benefits of this approach. This may be feasible in primary care, but requires an investment of organisation and of time.

Demonstration of skills

A variation on the group approach is an educational session that consists of a demonstration of skills delivered by either a practice member or an invited 'resource', such as a diabetes nurse specialist demonstrating blood glucose self-monitoring. It appears to be effective, although, as for most of the above methods, further research is needed.

Computer-assisted learning

Computer-assisted learning packages usually involve individual instruction, followed by tests of knowledge and understanding. The limited evidence suggests that they improve knowledge, may help glycaemic control and dietary habits, but have no demonstrable impact on weight loss. Such packages are not yet freely available in primary care. GP computer software has access to patient information systems, such as patient information leaflets (PILs), from which information leaflets can be printed off. Also, numerous websites provide high-quality information, such as the American National Institute of Health (NIH) and the diabetes organisations Diabetes UK and the ADA (see Chapter 14). However, these are not interactive and are unlikely to change behaviour.

Combination of teaching methods

In addition to the above specific approaches, the national guidelines discuss a combination of teaching methods that includes group and individual education, counselling, videotapes, 'empowerment' strategies, peer support and biofeedback-relaxation training. It is difficult to reach any definitive conclusions about the value of such combinations, as studies have used different combinations of the above and with little uniformity in the outcome measures. Some of these components are not easily available in primary care, but those involved in professional education already use a 'multi-faceted' approach that can be applied to patient education.

Patient activation–involvement approach

A patient activation–involvement approach takes a number of forms and uses a variety of strategies, and aims to encourage patients to become more involved in their care, particularly in decision-making. This is at the heart of NSF Standard 3, patient empowerment. It is a worthy aspiration and is at the centre of all patient encounters; evidence for its benefits in diabetic health education are limited to possible improvements in glycated haemoglobin and patient's knowledge, but no evidence indicates benefits in weight reduction, healthy eating, physical activity or lipid levels. It is not really a method, more an aim, as discussed at the start of Chapter 5.

Key Points of this Chapter

- Health education is more than imparting information, but is focussed often on modifying behaviour.

- Busy professionals can employ effective techniques that may alter a patient's motivation. Behavioural rather than didactic approaches are more likely to succeed.

- Evidence for the benefits of various educational approaches remains limited.

- The key educational messages are to stop smoking, to eat less and to exercise more.

REFERENCES

1 Kinmonth AL, Woodcock A, Griffin S, et al. Randomised controlled trial of patient centred care of diabetes in general practice: impact on current wellbeing and future disease risk. The diabetes care from diagnosis research team. BMJ 1998; **317**: 1202–1208.

2 Gask L, Usherwood T. ABC of psychological medicine: The consultation. BMJ 2002; **324**: 1567–1569.

3 Launer J. Narrative-based Primary Care: A Practical Guide. Oxford: Radcliffe Medical Press, 2002.

4 Prochaska JO, DiClemente CC. Stages of change in the modification of problem behaviors. Prog Behav Modif 1992; 28: 183–218.

5 Robertson N. A systematic approach to managing change. In: Baker R, Robertson N, Hearnshaw H, Eds. Implementing Change with Clinical Audit. Chichester: Wiley, 1979: 37–56.

6 Richardson P. Psychological treatments. In: Davies T, Craig TKJ (Eds). ABC of Mental Health. London: BMJ Books, 1998.

7 Enright J. Fortnightly review: Cognitive behaviour therapy – clinical applications. BMJ 1997; **314**: 1811–1823.

8 Stewart MA. Effective physician–patient communication and health outcomes: a review. CMAJ 1995; **152**: 1423–1433.

9 Scottish Intercollegiate Guidelines Network. Management of Diabetes: A National Clinical Guideline (Number 55). Edinburgh: SIGN Executive, Royal College of Physicians, 2001. Online: www.sign.ac.uk

10 McIntosh A, Hutchinson A, Home PD, et al. Clinical Guidelines for Type 2 Diabetes: Blood glucose management. Sheffield: ScHARR, University of Sheffield, 2002. Online: http://www.shef.ac.uk/guidelines/

11 Albright A, Franz M, Hornsby G, et al. American College of Sports Medicine Position Stand. Exercise and type 2 diabetes. Med Sci Sports Exerc 2000; **32**: 1345–1360.

CHAPTER THIRTEEN

Measuring Performance: Audit

What Is Audit?

Professor Robin Fraser has provided an excellent definition of audit that is particularly relevant to primary care: 'Audit is the process of looking critically and systematically at our own professional activities with a view to improving personal/practice performance and the quality and/or cost effectiveness of patient care'.[1] The aims of audit in primary care should be:[2]

- To identify and to use methods to improve the quality of care;
- To assess one's own performance in a systematic way;
- To ensure that resources are used effectively; and
- To facilitate education and training among doctors and their practice staff.

Guidance for undertaking clinical audit has been set out in the book *Principles for Best Practice in Clinical Audit*, published in March 2002.[3] In addition, Quality Indicators for Diabetes Services (QUIDS) has developed an audit methodology 'appropriate for measuring the clinical quality performance of population based (primary and secondary care) routine, continuing diabetes care'. The final report commissioned by NICE, Diabetes UK and the NHS Executive Northwest, is now available[4] and compliments the Diabetes Information Strategy (see Chapter 5).

Stages of Clinical Audit, as Applied to Diabetic Care

The process can be divided into five stages, although not all of the steps in each stage are needed in every diabetic audit:

- Prepare for audit;
- Select criteria;
- Measure performance;
- Make improvements;
- Sustain improvement.

Prepare for audit

The steps involved include:

- Involve users (staff, patients) in the process.
- Topic selection, influenced by the team's interests and requirements, and by clinical governance considerations (local and NSF). *Table 13.1* suggests aspects of diabetic care that may be suitable for audit. If using the periodic review (see *Table 8.1*), then the audit could follow the sequence in *Table 13.2*, discussed in more detail below.
- Define the purpose of the audit ('to improve, to enhance, to ensure or to change').

- Provide the necessary structures so that audit is an integral part of the team's work.
- Identify and provide the skills, people (including training) and resources required.

Select criteria

Criteria

Criteria are explicit statements that define what is being measured and represent elements of care that can be measured. 'Valid' criteria should be based upon evidence (justifiable) and related to aspects of care important to the team and/or patient. Criteria can be classified into three groups:

- Structure (what you need);
- Process (what you do);
- Outcome of care (what you expect).

Criteria should be justified by the highest available level of evidence (see Chapter 14). New methods of selecting criteria that may become relevant to diabetes care are *benchmarking* (compare and set target levels of performance in comparison to other organisations) and *integrated care pathways* (describe explicitly the expected processes of care at each stage of man-

Table 13.1. Aspects of diabetic care suitable for audit[5]	
Criteria group	Suitable examples
1. Structures (resources required)	*Availability of specific items* (e.g., a large sphygmomanometer cuff, protocol) *Availability of specific facilities* (e.g., dark room for fundoscopy, educational resources, protected time for reviews) *Practice diabetic register*: does the practice's prevalence equal the local estimate? What is the ethnicity of the diabetic population? *Training* for team members
2. Processes (actions and decisions taken by practitioners together with users)	*Appointments* – waiting times and default rate *Record* in the notes of checks of parameters for periodic review agreed in the practice protocol *Uptake* of influenza vaccination in type 2 patients *Information* given to patients as part of their education
3. Outcomes (measures of the physical or behavioural response to an intervention, reported health status or level of knowledge and satisfaction); some of these can be used as performance indicators to measure progress in: • medication and diet; • implementing the NSF; • meeting the St. Vincent Task Force objectives	*Results of parameters* checked (e.g., levels of blood pressure, HbA1c, frequency of hypoglycaemic episodes) *Complications*, such as retinopathy or registrable blindness, nephropathy or renal failure (requiring renal replacement therapy), lower limb amputations *Significant events* (e.g., referrals, emergency hospital admissions, deaths, incidence of myocardial infarction) *Levels of patient knowledge* about self-monitoring *Days off work* *Quality of life*

agement for a particular condition for which there is an established routine with little variation – the measurements are integrated into the medical record).

Standards
Standards are the percentage of events that should comply with the criterion.[6] If standards are set, they need to be agreed by the practice team, to be based upon relevant high-quality research evidence (if available) and to be realistic (current targets for glycaemic control, lipids and blood pressure are not always attainable). As the aim of the audit is to improve care, standards may be set just above the predicted level of performance.

Measure performance
Good performance of this stage is facilitated by a good practice organisation (see Chapter 5). The steps involved include:
- Planning data collection;
- Identifying the study population;
- Handling data;
- Analysing data;
- Presenting findings;
- Ethical and legal implications.

Planning data collection
The team needs to agree about the group of patients to be studied, the time period over which the criteria apply and the type of data analysis to be used. Consultation with those involved with the aspect of care being studied is essential. These measures increase precision and ensure the collection of only essential data.

Identifying the study population
An accurate, up-to-date diabetic register simplifies matters. If the relevant morbidity data are recorded manually, it may not be feasible or practical to include every patient in the audit; representative sampling should be done using a statistically valid method (outside statistical advice may be helpful; see also *Principles for Best Practice in Clinical Audit* for guidance[3]).

Handling data
The methods used depend upon how diabetic information is recorded in the practice. Audit is facilitated if data are recorded accurately, with the coding agreed and in the most retrievable form. The existing record and information systems, particularly if the patient records are electronic, may be adequate to provide the necessary data. MIQUEST is software that uses health-query language to access, aggregate and analyse data held in GP computer systems. It is valuable to check a sample of the manual records (if they are used in any way) to assess the completeness of electronic data capture. If there is a substantial amount of 'missing' data, a trawl through the written notes and any other data sources will be needed. The protocol for data extraction should be clear and agreed. Data may be extracted onto agreed standard forms (the Clinical Governance Research and Development Unit package provides an example) or entered directly into a computer database. Data extraction from manual records is a tedious, time-consuming process, so it may be considered 'fair play' to divide this task among the clinical members of the team.

Table 13.2. Audit example for diabetic care: evaluating the periodic review

Aim

To improve the quality of checks undertaken as part of the periodic diabetic review

Review criteria to be selected

These are the measurements in the known practice diabetic population of the frequency of checks, the proportion of abnormal findings and whether appropriate action is taken for each component listed in *Table 8.1*. When analysing the periodic review, it may be helpful also to collect demographic data, including age, sex, year of diagnosis, check the patient is on the practice diabetic register, venue of delivery of diabetic care (i.e., practice, hospital or shared)

Justification of criteria

The above criteria are the contents of the practice diabetic protocol and will provide factual evidence of the quality of diabetic care being delivered in the practice. The definition of abnormality and the intervention that follows form part of the protocol

Standards to be set

Standards to be set depend upon the best evidence from other audits or upon a consensus among the team:
1. For each criterion, the proportion of type 2 patients being checked;
2. For each criterion, the proportion of abnormal findings depends upon the criterion (e.g., more type 2 patients will have a raised HbA1c or blood pressure than albuminuria);
3. For each abnormal finding that appropriate action is taken

Data collection

If manual, team members to extract data from a statistically significant (95% confidence interval) sample of notes on an agreed recording form; if electronic, use appropriate search tool

Results

Presented in a tabular form:
1. General morbidity data:
   - Practice size, age and sex distribution;
   - Diabetic study population – numbers, age and sex distribution, duration of diabetes (bands), venue of diabetic care
2. Data for each criterion:
   - Numbers checked;
   - Proportion of checks with abnormal findings;
   - Proportion of abnormal findings in which appropriate action is taken

Discussion of results

Performance against standards; if standards were not reached, why?

Negotiated plans to improve performance against review criteria

Agree specific tasks for each member of the team, and include a timetable for the next data collection with revised standards

Analysing data

Data analysis can range from a simple calculation of percentages to more sophisticated statistical techniques. Simple methods are usually preferable.

Presenting findings

The findings should be presented clearly, with the appropriate use of graphs and tables. It is common for the standard of performance against the agreed criteria to be worse than expected or hoped for. This justifies undertaking the audit! The practice team then needs to analyse the reason(s) for this shortfall, and so to improve the standard of performance in the future.

Ethical and legal implications

Data collection may have ethical and legal implications, particularly related to confidentiality. The Data Protection Act 1998[7] must be respected. The professional bodies, the General Medical Council[8] and the Nursing and Midwifery Council have issued guidance in this area.

Make improvements

Practices that have in place the structure to support efforts to make improvements, including personal professional development, are at an advantage. The likelihood of improved performance in the future will be much greater if any action plan:

- Is negotiated and agreed within the practice team and by its key members, a process in which barriers to change need to be identified and tackled (the use of the trans-theoretical model, discussed in Chapter 12, also applies to changing professional's behaviour);[9]
- Involves teamwork and ownership of the planned changes; and
- Is specific, with clearly defined tasks and accountability for each participant.

Action plans should include a timetable for the next data collection and revised standards for performance against each criterion.

Sustain improvement

Sustaining improvement is an extension of the structures and processes by which improvements are made. Lessons learned from audits, critical events and high-quality evidence-based guidance need to be incorporated into daily work. Regular learning activities that improve the knowledge and skills of the team in a focussed way, based upon individual and team needs, should be one of a practice's essential activities. Much of the clinical governance literature cited above and in the introduction discusses these issues.

Key Points of this Chapter

- Audit can improve care if undertaken in a systematic way with sensible recommendations for change.
- Audit topics can include aspects of structure, process and outcome of interest to the team, such as the periodic review.

REFERENCES

1 Fraser RC. Medical audit in general practice. *Trainee* 1982; **2**: 142–145.

2 Leicestershire Medical Audit Advisory Group. *A Guide to Audit.* Leicester: Leicestershire MAAG, 1993.

3 NICE, Commission for Health Improvement, Royal College of Nursing, University of Leicester. *Principles for Best Practice in Clinical Audit.* Oxford: Radcliffe Medical Press, March 2002. Online: http://www.nice.org.uk

4 NICE, Diabetese UK and the NHS Executive Northwest. *Quality Indicators for Diabetes Services (QUIDS). Final Report of a Development Project Commissioned by NICE, Diabetese UK and the NHS Executive Northwest.* Online: http://www.quids.org.uk/

5 Griffin SJ, Kinmonth A-L. The management of diabetes by general practitioners and shared care. In: Pickup JC, Williams G, Eds. *Textbook of Diabetes*, 2nd Edn. Oxford: Blackwell Scientific, 1997: Ch 80.

6 Baker R, Fraser RC. Development of audit criteria: linking guidelines and assessment of quality. *BMJ* 1995; **31**: 370–373.

7 HMSO. *Data Protection Act 1998.* Online: www.hmso.gov.uk/acts/acts1998/19980029.htm

8 General Medical Council. *Confidentiality: Protecting and Providing Information.* London: General Medical Council, 2000.

9 Robertson N, Baker R, Hearnshaw H. Changing the clinical behaviour of doctors – a psychological framework. *Qual Health Care* 1996; **5**: 51–54.

CHAPTER FOURTEEN

Evidence-Based Diabetic Care

This book is a practical guide, so it is not intended to cover in depth every aspect of type 2 diabetes. Furthermore, parts of the book will eventually become out of date as a result of the publication of new research and yet more official guidelines. Therefore, the reader may find this chapter a helpful guide on how to begin to obtain further information and to evaluate it. Electronic addresses do change, but those listed below and elsewhere in this book are correct at the time of writing.

Evidenced-Based Medicine: A Very Brief Overview

Basic concepts

Optimal patient care requires practitioners to base their decisions about intervention upon the best available evidence. Practitioners of evidence-based medicine (EBM) argue that effective clinicians:

1 Ask focussed answerable clinical questions in terms of the:
   - Patient or problem;
   - Intervention;
   - Comparison intervention, if appropriate;
   - Outcome.
2 Search the literature effectively for the best evidence.
3 Assess critically the quality of this evidence. When evaluating a study, it may be useful to ask:
   - Is the population recruited for a study representative of what most GPs see?
   - Can a GP practice reliably and safely carry out the studied intervention and any associated activities without detriment to the patient or the practice's total portfolio of professional services?
   - Does the presentation of randomised controlled trials (RCTs) conform to the CONSORT guidelines?[1]
   - Is the outcome's endpoint both measurable in and relevant to primary care?
   Beware that the interpretation of large and important studies, such as UKPDS and HOPE, is not without controversy.
4 Integrate this evidence into a management plan, as negotiated with the patient.

Evidence base for recommendations

It is now common practice for the guidance documents published by authoritative bodies, such as NSF, NICE and SIGN, to indicate the type of evidence used to support their recommendations. The classification and definitions of these types of evidence originate from the

Table 14.1. Levels of evidence (combining definitions used by NSF and NICE)

Level	Type of evidence
1a	Meta-analyses, systematic reviews of randomised control trials
1b	At least one randomised control trial
2a	Systematic reviews of case-control or cohort studies (without randomisation)
2b	At least one case-control or cohort study
3	Nonanalytical studies (e.g., case reports, case series)
4	Expert opinion (in the absence of any of the above)

US Agency for Health Care Policy and Research (see *Table 14.1*). All bodies agree upon the main levels (1 to 4 in *Table 14.1*), but may vary upon how many divisions to include at each level. Obviously, level 1 evidence using RCTs carries the greatest weight.

Many of the documents issued for guidance by expert bodies use a grading scheme for their recommendations, as summarised in *Table 14.2*.

Evidence-based medicine resources

It is far beyond the scope of this book to describe how to carry out EBM. The two following books are excellent guides for beginners:

- Sackett DL, Strauss SE, Richardson WS, *et al. Evidence-Based Medicine: How to Practice and Teach EBM* , 2nd Edn. Edinburgh: Churchill Livingstone, 2000.
- Greenhalgh T. *How to Read a Paper: The Basics of Evidence Based Medicine*, 2nd Edn. London: BMJ Publishing Group, 2000.

The following electronic EBM resources (not a comprehensive list) may be valuable as a starting point:

- *Finding answers to questions in EBM* is an excellent Norwegian site (in English) for beginners, and it has useful links: http://www.uib.no/isf/people/atle/ebm.htm
- *Netting the Evidence Guide* on: http://www.sheffield.ac.uk/~scharr/ir/netting

Table 14.2. Grades of recommendations[2]

Grade	Evidence used
A	Directly based upon level 1 evidence
B	Directly based upon level 2 evidence, or extrapolated recommendation from level 1 evidence
C	Directly based upon level 3 evidence, or extrapolated recommendation from level 1 or 2 evidence
D	Directly based upon level 4 evidence, or extrapolated recommendation from level 1, 2 or 3 evidence

Resources: Where to Start Looking

The lists of further sources of information listed below are daunting, but I recommend that the reader begins at:

- The Scottish Intercollegiate Guidelines Network (SIGN) and the American Diabetes Association (ADA) for guidelines;
- MacKinnon M. *Providing Diabetes Care in General Practice: A Practical Guide for the Primary Care Team*, 4th Edn. London: Class Publishing, 2002;
- PubMed and Cochrane for up to date medical literature and reviews.

The following lists should be regarded as starting points. Journals and electronic resources are more likely to be up to date.

Books or booklets

- Diabetes UK. *Recommendations for the Management of Diabetes in Primary Care*, 3rd Edn. London: Diabetes UK, 2000;
- Department of Health. *National Service Framework for Diabetes: Standards*. London: HMSO, 2001;
- Department of Health. *National Service Framework for Diabetes: Delivery Strategy*. London: HMSO, 2002;
- Krentz AJ, Bailey CJ. *Type 2 Diabetes in Practice*. London: Royal Society of Medicine Press Ltd, 2001;
- MacKinnon M. *Providing Diabetes Care in General Practice: A Practical Guide for the Primary Care Team*, 4th Edn. London: Class Publishing, 2002;
- Pickup JC, Williams G, Eds. *Textbook of Diabetes*, 2nd Edn. Oxford: Blackwell Scientific, 1997.
- Williams B. *Diabetes and Hypertension: A Fatal Attraction Explained*. Beckenham: Publishing Initiatives Books, 1996.

Journals

Practical Diabetes International is published every two months and is excellent, from PMH Publications, PO BOX 100, Chichester, West Sussex, PO18 8HD, who mail it free on request to health care professionals.

Diabetes Digest is also very useful for keeping up to date with diabetes literature. It is published quarterly in the UK for health care professionals with an interest in diabetes and can be obtained from SB Communications Group, 15 Mandeville Courtyard, 142 Battersea Park Road, London SW11 4NB (telephone 020 7627 1510; e-mail: info@sbcommunications-group.com).

Important research and reviews about diabetes may be published in eminent peer-reviewed journals with wide circulation, such as the *British Medical Journal, Lancet* or *New England Journal of Medicine*, or those with specialist interest, such as *Diabetes Care, Diabetic Medicine* or *Diabetologica*. These are either available on subscription or are held in any self-respecting hospital postgraduate library.

Electronic resources

With the proliferation of electronic resources, it may seem a self-defeating exercise to produce a printed book. Traditional textbooks fail frequently to incorporate newly published research. Furthermore, textbooks may lack specific references, selected according to explicit principles of evidence, to support their declarations about diagnosis and management. However, the production of this book is proof of the author's and his publisher's belief in the value of a practical and organised overview of a complex field in an accessible medium.

Electronic evidence databases, available either via the Internet or on CD-ROM, are regarded as being better able to overcome the above drawbacks. No single database will address all needs. A comprehensive search needs to choose an effective strategy to look at several appropriate databases. Try contacting the local postgraduate medical library to cultivate the medical librarian and to book a training session: it is well worth it! Another invaluable benefit of contacting the local postgraduate library is to obtain a personal ATHENS (Access to Higher Education via NISS Authentication System) username and password, which allows access to many remote electronic resources, such as the *Cochrane Library*. The following databases are useful:

1 Many, but not all, medical articles are indexed in the massive *Medline* database, compiled by the National Library of Medicine in the USA. There is no filtering on the original Medline, so each article needs to be evaluated critically. Free access to Medline has been available since 1997 via PubMed, online: http://www.ncbi.nih.gov/entrez/query.fcgi
   PubMed has other useful features:[3]
   - LinkOut includes full text articles, biological databases, consumer health information and research tools;
   - ClinicalTrials.gov is a database that provides current information about clinical research studies;
   - A new 'Clinical Queries' feature filter references, and aims to retrieve systematic reviews and meta-analysis studies for a specific search topic.
   The British Library can provide more information about lesser known PubMed features, online: www.bl.uk/services/information/blmedline.html

2 The *Cochrane Library* is a collection of databases, updated quarterly, that includes systematic reviews and registers of controlled trials. It is not yet comprehensive, but it is user-friendly and expanding rapidly. Many researchers now favour *Cochrane* when starting a literature search. It can be obtained on a subscription basis, either on CD-ROM or via the Internet, from Update Software Ltd., Summertown, Pavilion, Middle Way, Oxford, OX2 7LG. Tel 01865 513902 or Web: http://www.update-software.com/cochrane/order.htm or e-mail: info@update.co.uk. The *Cochrane Database of Systematic Reviews* is an important information source for the effectiveness of treatments. It is available free to NHS staff via the knowledge section of the National Electronic Library of Health (NeLH) http://www.nelh.nhs.uk/ and the abstracts are free to all via: http://www.update-software.com/cochrane/abstract.htm

3 The University of York's NHS Centre for Reviews and Dissemination (CRD) maintains several free related databases (online: http://agatha.york.ac.uk/welcome.htm):
   - *DARE* (Database of Abstracts of Reviews of Effect);
   - *NHS EED* (the NHS economic evaluation database);
   - *HTA* (health technology assessment).

4 *EmBase* (online: http://www.embase.bids.ac.uk/embase) focuses on drugs, but requires an ATHENS-authenticated username and password for access.

5 NeLH is available free to NHS staff via the NHSNet (online: http://www.nelh.nhs.uk/). It has other useful features:

- Research Findings Register;
- A dedicated web site for health care professionals looking after patients with diabetes (online: http://cebmh.warne.ox.ac.uk/diabetes/professional/);

6 TRIP is a free database that searches over 55 sites of high-quality medical information (online: http://www.tripdatabase.com/).

7 A number of excellent resources with good links enable the user to access a wide range of useful high-quality information on the Internet:

- The North Glasgow University Hospitals NHS Trust has an excellent electronic library with useful links (online: http://www.northglashealthinfo.org.uk);
- DiabetesMonitor.com is another American website for both professionals and patients (online: http://www.diabetesmonitor.com/);
- The National Institute of Diabetes and Digestive Kidney Diseases is part of the American National Institute of Health (online: http://www.niddk.nih.gov/);
- The Tayside Regional Diabetes Network is a useful resource with professional guidance (via the NHSNet) and downloadable patient leaflets (online: http://www.diabetes-healthnet.ac.uk).

Organisations

Many organisations have their own websites with useful information:

- The American Diabetic Association publishes comprehensive and referenced clinical practice recommendations that are up-dated annually (online: http://www.diabetes.org);
- Diabetes UK, formerly the British Diabetic Association, caters not only for health care professionals, but also for patients and other interested lay people, at 10 Parkway, London NW1 7AA, telephone (020) 7424 1000. GPs and practice nurses can join the Primary Care section (online: http://www.diabetes.org.uk);
- The Department of Health, for finding official documents (online: http://www.doh.gov.uk);
- National Institute for Clinical Excellence, for guidelines, particularly on new treatments (online: http://www.nice.org.uk);
- The Scottish Intercollegiate Guidelines Network published in November 2001 its own guidelines for the management of diabetes. Their evidence base is very well set out and they carry an extensive list of references. They can be downloaded from the SIGN website (online: http://www.sign.ac.uk/);
- Clinical Governance Research and Development Unit, Department of General Practice and Primary Health Care, University of Leicester, Leicester General Hospital, Gwendolen Road, Leicester LE5 4PW (online: http://www.le.ac.uk/cgrdu/);
- The University of Warwick's *Warwick Diabetes Care* was launched in November 2000. It is an extremely useful point of contact for all providers of diabetic care through educational courses, support of diabetes research and practical resources and links. It can be contacted via telephone (024) 7657 2958, e-mail: diabetes@warwick.ac.uk or website (online: http://www.diabetescare.warwick.ac.uk).

Key Points of this Chapter

- Optimal patient care requires the practitioner to base decisions about intervention upon the best-available evidence.

- With such a wide range of written and electronic information available, a clear effective strategy needs to be used to obtain useful information.

- Several excellent websites are now available, particularly via the National electronic library for Health

REFERENCES

1 Altman DG, Schulz KF, Moher D, *et al*; CONSORT GROUP (Consolidated Standards of Reporting Trials). The revised CONSORT statement for reporting randomized trials: explanation and elaboration. *Ann Intern Med* 2001; 134: 663–694.

2 Eccles M, Freemantle N, Mason J. North of England Evidence Based Guidance Development Project: guideline for angiotensin converting enzyme inhibitors in primary care management of adults with symptomatic heart failure. *BMJ* 1998; **316**: 1369–1375.

3 Kotzin S. Medline and PubMed will be able to synthesise clinical data (letter). *BMJ* 2002; **324**: 791.

Appendix 1

Table A.1. Correlation between HbA1c level and mean plasma glucose levels*

HbA1c (%)	Mean plasma glucose level (mmol/l)
6	7.5
7	9.5
8	11.5
9	13.5
10	15.5
11	17.5
12	19.5

*Rohlfing CL, Wiedmeyer HM, Little RR, et al. Defining the relationship between plasma glucose and HbA1c: analysis of glucose profiles and HbA1c in the Diabetes Control and Complications Trial. *Diabetes Care* 2002; 25: 275–278.

Index

Table A.1. New GMS contract indicators for diabetes and where they are discussed herein

Indicator	Points	Maximum threshold	Where discussed
DM7: The percentage of patients with diabetes in whom the last HbA1c is 10 or less (or equivalent test / reference range depending on local laboratory) in last 15 months	11	85%	Chapter 8: pp. 63–64. See also Chapter 7 sections on diet and treatment
DM8: The percentage of diabetic patients who have a record of retinal screening in the previous 15 months	5	90%	Chapter 8: pp. 85–89
DM9: The percentage of patients with diabetes with a record of presence or absence of peripheral pulses in the previous 15 months	3	90%	Chapter 8: pp. 80–85
DM10: The percentage of patients with diabetes with a record of neuropathy testing in the previous 15 months	3	90%	Chapter 8: pp. 80–85
DM11: The percentage of patients with diabetes who have a record of the blood pressure in the past 15 months	3	90%	Chapter 8: pp. 69–75
DM12: The percentage of patients with diabetes in whom the last blood pressure is 148/85 or less	17	55%	Chapter 8: pp. 69–75
DM13: The percentage of patients with diabetes who have a record of micro-albuminuria testing in the previous 15 months (exception reporting for patients with proteinuria)	3	90%	Chapter 8: pp. 88–90
DM14: The percentage of patients with diabetes who have a record of serum creatinine testing in the previous 15 months	3	90%	Chapter 8: pp. 90–91
DM15: The percentage of patients with diabetes with proteinuria or micro-albuminuria who are treated with ACE inhibitors (or A2 antagonists)	3	70%	Chapter 8: pp. 73–74
DM16: The percentage of patients with diabetes who have a record of total cholesterol in the previous 15 months	3	90%	Chapter 8: pp. 76–80
DM17: The percentage of patients with diabetes whose last measured total cholesterol within previous 15 months is 5 or less	6	60%	Chapter 8: pp. 76–80. See also Chapter 7 section on diet
DM18: The percentage of patients with diabetes who have had influenza immunisation in the preceding 1 September to 31 March	3	85%	Chapter 5

ADDENDUM

New GMS contract indicators for diabetes

Since this book went to press, the new GMS contract has been published. One of its main features is to link a proportion of a practice's remuneration to the quality of services it delivers in several clinical areas, such as diabetes. Frameworks have set up, whereby points are awarded for achievement against a number of indicators (weighted differently depending upon the workload implications) in a direct linear relationship between the minimum, set at 25% for clinical indicators, and the maximum, set at a practically achievable level. The following table lists each diabetes indicator, its points and maximum threshold, and the section of this book where the topic is discussed.

Table A.1. New GMS contract indicators for diabetes and where they are discussed herein (All minimum thresholds are 25%.)

Indicator	Points	Maximum threshold	Where discussed
DM1: The practice can produce a register of all patients with diabetes mellitus	6	Not applicable	Chapter 5: organisation
DM2: The percentage of patients with diabetes whose notes record BMI in the previous 12 months	3	90%	Chapter 8: review p. 75–76
DM3: The percentage of patients with diabetes in whom there is a record of smoking status in the previous 15 months except those who have never smoked where smoking status should be recorded once	3	90%	Chapter 8: pp. 67 & 69
DM4: The percentage of patients with diabetes who smoke and whose notes contain a record that smoking cessation advice has been offered in the last 15 months	5	90%	Chapter 8: pp. 67 & 69
DM5: The percentage of diabetic patients who have a record of HbA1c or equivalent in the previous 15 months	3	90%	Chapter 8: pp. 63–64
The percentage of patients with whom the last HbA1c is 7.4 equivalent test / reference on local laboratory) in	16	50%	Chapter 8: pp. 63–64. See also Chapter 7 sections on diet and treatment